Commissioning Editor: Ellen Green
Development Editor: Joan Morrison
Project Manager: Emma Riley
Senior Designer: Sarah Russell
Illustration Manager: Bruce Hogarth

Pass the Preregistration Pharmacy Exam

Chi-Loon Cheung
MPharm (Hons) MRPharms
Locum Pharmacist
London, UK

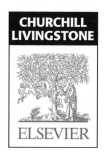

EDINBURGH   LONDON   NEW YORK   OXFORD   PHILADELPHIA   ST LOUIS   SYDNEY   TORONTO 2006

CHURCHILL
LIVINGSTONE
ELSEVIER

First published 2006

ISBN 0 443 100845

*British Library Cataloguing
in Publication Data*
A catalogue record for this book is available from the British Library.

*Library of Congress Cataloging
in Publication Data*
A catalog record for this book is available from the Library of Congress.

Notice
Knowledge and best practice in this field are constantly changing. As new research and experience broaden our knowledge, changes in practice, treatment and drug therapy may become necessary or appropriate. Readers are advised to check the most current information provided (i) on procedures featured or (ii) by the manufacturer of each product to be administered, to verify the recommended dose or formula, the method and duration of administration, and contraindications. It is the responsibility of the practitioner, relying on their own experience and knowledge of the patient, to make diagnoses, to determine dosages and the best treatment for each individual patient, and to take all appropriate safety precautions. To the fullest extent of the law, neither the publisher nor the author assumes any liability for any injury and/or damage to persons or property arising out of, or related to, any use of the material contained in this book.

The Publisher

The
Publisher's
policy is to use
**paper manufactured
from sustainable forests**

Printed in China

Preface

The Royal Pharmaceutical Society preregistration membership exam is unlike any examination that you may have previously encountered. All the years of dedication and hard work amassed during the MPharm degree course and the preregistration year will be tested, thereby determining whether one can practice as a pharmacist.

Recent results have shown that between 80 and 95% of candidates pass the membership exam. At first glance, this gives the impression that the exam is relatively easy. Yet this could not be further from the truth. A pass mark of 70% is required in both the main assessments (open- and closed-book) and the newly introduced calculations paper. Another way of looking at this is that an A grade is required to pass the exam!

The preregistration exam in essence is an assessment of competence in that it asks whether the person sitting the exam is ready to take on the responsibilities of being a pharmacist. For this reason, the preregistration year should be taken seriously as many of the answers for the exam will be based on the experience gained during training.

The approach to taking the preregistration exam is to learn and understand the working practices of pharmacy. In meeting this objective, you should ensure that all training competencies are fulfilled and think about why a pharmacist would use them. In addition, all available learning resources should be used, including asking pharmacists about their practice methods.

Passing the preregistration exam is a huge achievement which not only allows membership to a proud and noble profession but also marks the beginning of an interesting and varied career.

How to use this book

The preregistration exam tests five key areas of practice, which are:

1. Clinical pharmacy and therapeutics: examines knowledge about the use and effects of medicines;
2. Pharmacy practice: assesses aspects of pharmacy practice;

3. Pharmacy law and ethics: assesses knowledge of legislation and practice applied to pharmacy practice;
4. Responding to symptoms: determines whether the candidate can diagnose and treat minor ailments;
5. Calculations: the manipulation of mathematical techniques and accuracy required by a pharmacist.

Each chapter covers one of the above areas of practice and summarises information all preregistration candidates are expected to know. Following the summaries are questions examining the particular area of practice, set out in the style of the preregistration exam. Fully explained answers, with the appropriate references, are given at the back of the book. The answers have been written in a style that allows them to read as revision notes, without the need to refer back to the question.

This book is not intended to be a comprehensive guide to the practice of pharmacy. It should be used to identify any areas of weakness, and as an opportunity to improve your examination technique for the actual preregistration exam.

Acknowledgements

I would like to thank all those who have helped in producing this book, especially Penny Lewis (University of Manchester) and Alicia Salisbury (Walsall Manor Hospital NHS Trust) for the assistance and information they provided when this book was in the planning stage. Additional thanks are due to all the pharmacy staff at Birmingham Children's Hospital NHS Trust for laying the foundations of my pharmacy career.

I am extremely grateful for the inspiration and advice continually provided by Professor Kevin Taylor and Dr Abdul Basit (both at the School of Pharmacy, London). Thanks are also due to the editorial staff of Elsevier Publishers for their guidance, in particular Ellen Green who commissioned the project, and also Joan Morrison.

Finally, I would like to thank my family for their loving support, with particular mention to my brother, Seau-Tak, whose idea gave birth to this project.

Chi-Loon Cheung
London

Contents

1 The Preregistration Examination

The preregistration exam has three components:

- Closed book paper: 90 questions in 90 minutes; tests fundamental knowledge and understanding of professional aspects of pharmacy practice
- Open book paper: 60 questions in 90 minutes; assesses the ability to gain appropriate and accurate information from allowed reference sources ('BNF', 'Drug Tariff' and 'Medicine, Ethics and Practice: a Guide for Pharmacists')
- Calculations paper: 20 question in 60 minutes; assesses ability to obtain accurate values by the manipulation of mathematical techniques.

All three papers are sat on the same day, with most students attempting their first sitting in late June or early July. (The re-sit exam is held in late September.) Exam day consists of two distinct sessions: the closed book paper being in the morning, and the open book and calculations papers are taken together in the afternoon. Lunch immediately follows the morning session and lasts for 2 hours; it is highly recommended that students eat something and relax during the break, as the afternoon session can be mentally and physically exhausting.

To pass the exam, an overall pass mark of 70% or over must be gained from the combined answers from the open and closed book papers, and a separate pass mark of 70% or over must be obtained in the calculations paper. Failure to pass the combined papers and the calculation will result in a failed exam attempt.

Further information regarding the open book references

The specified references to be used in the open book paper are the 'British National Formulary' (BNF), 'Medicine, Ethics and Practice: a Guide for Pharmacists', and the 'Drug Tariff'. It is not of great importance to remember the vast quantities of information held within the open book references, rather that you know which book is the most appropriate to use for a particular area of pharmacy. Questions in the open book paper are meant to reflect situations occurring in the practice of pharmacy. An alternative interpretation is that anything can be (and usually is) questioned about the information contained in these references.

It is imperative to read through all the open book reference books at an early stage of employment, preferably within the first 3 months of starting. In doing so, there should be plenty of time to work through any difficulties that you may have concerning the information contained in BNF, Medicine, Ethics and Practice: a Guide for Pharmacists or Drug Tariff. Hence, a greater appreciation and understanding is developed regarding pharmacy practice, which translates into more confidence for the preregistration exam.

You should practise using, at every opportunity, the editions required for your exam sitting. This will enable you to become familiar with the type of information contained within each book, and it makes the books easier to use (new books tend to be stiff and pages tend to stick together).

Examination regulations allow the following personal additions to be made to the specified reference sources:

- sections of text may be highlighted or underlined;
- 'tags' or 'flags' may be used to identify particular pages (see recommended pages to tab);
- short notes may be written into the page margins as long as they are relevant to the text;
- it is forbidden to insert 'post-it' notes or pages; reference books are checked by the examination invigilators to ensure that there is no excessive annotation of notes.

Open book reference: British National Formulary (BNF)

The BNF, contrary to popular opinion, is not recognised by the Medicines Act 1968 as an official reference book. Nevertheless, it is a very useful resource for all healthcare professionals and every preregistration student should consider it as his or her bible. The bulk of the book is structured into chapters detailing drug use of main organ systems, with disease states dividing each chapter. The beginning of the book describes prescribing guidance and the emergency treating of poisoning; whereas interactions and drug use in impaired organ function are detailed at the end of the book. See Tables 1.1 and 1.2 for exam tips.

Open book reference: Medicine, Ethics and Practice: a Guide for Pharmacists

This book offers guidance on the conduct of pharmacists and how pharmacy should be practised. Some words of warning: law and ethics

Table 1.1 Main areas of the BNF required for the preregistration exam

- Prescribing guidance (in particular the section on prescribing in palliative care)
- Guidance on adverse reactions to drugs
- Emergency treatment of poisoning
- Chapter introductions of each organ system
- Guidance notes on drug use of each disease state
- Appendices
- CSM and BNF advices and warnings

Table 1.2 Suggested BNF pages to tab

- Chapter opening for main organ systems
- Equivalent doses of oral morphine and parenteral diamorphine (part of prescribing in palliative care)
- Equivalent doses of oral corticosteroids
- Potencies of topical corticosteroids
- Appendices
- Dental and nurse practitioners' formularies
- Index

can be a very trying (i.e. dull) topic to study but you must persevere as a significant proportion of this book is examined. There should be no need to supplement the information content in this publication. See Tables 1.3 and 1.4 for exam tips.

Open book reference: Drug Tariff

This is a monthly publication from the Department of Health and is sent to all contractors of the NHS. It details how the services are to be reimbursed and remunerated. An awareness of the contents of this book is all that is required for the preregistration exam. See Table 1.5 for exam tips.

Question styles encountered in the preregistration exam

The overall objective of the exam is to test how the candidate will approach situations they may encounter during the practice of pharmacy. Hence, questions are designed to demonstrate analytical and evaluation skills, comprehension and knowledge. Four different types of multiple-choice questions (MCQs) make up the preregistration exam. Not answering enough questions is the reason most cited as the cause for failing. MCQs are not negatively marked; therefore, if you do not know an answer just guess! Examples of the different MCQ

Table 1.3 Main areas of Medicine, Ethics and Practice: a Guide for Pharmacists required for the preregistration exam

- Prescribing and supply of medicinal products
- Emergency supplies of POMs
- Labelling of medicinal products
- Controlled drugs
- Non-medicinal poisons
- CHIP Regulations 2002
- Methylated spirits
- Prescribing and dispensing of veterinary drugs
- Duties and responsibility of pharmacists
- Continued professional development (CPD)
- Audits
- Clinical governance
- Guidance on the provision of pharmaceutical services
- Responsibilities of the superintendent pharmacist

Table 1.4 Suggested Medicine, Ethics and Practice: a Guide for Pharmacists pages to tab

- Contents page
- Meaning of retail sale and wholesale dealing
- Prescribing and labelling of POMs
- Emergency supplies of POMs
- Ophthalmic opticians: sale or supply
- Ambulance paramedics: administration
- Table summarising legal requirements of controlled drugs
- Start of alphabetical list of medicines for human use
- Table of aspirin legal status
- Table of paracetamol legal status
- Non-medicinal poisons
- Start of alphabetical list of non-medicinal poisons
- CHIP regulations 2002 (i.e. chemicals)
- Methylated spirits
- Start of alphabetical list of medicines for veterinary use
- Start of 'Part 2: standards of professional performance' (this marks the position for the responsibilities and provisions of service by a pharmacist and the duties of a superintendent pharmacist)
- Guidance on good practice
- Improving the quality of pharmacy practices (this marks the position for clinical governance and CPD)
- Index

Table 1.5 Suggested Drug Tariff pages to tab

- Contents page
- Part II: calculation of payments
- Part II: zero discount lists
- Part III A: professional fees
- Part VI A: additional professional fees
- Part VIII: basic prices for generic medication
- Part IX A: bandages
- Part IX A: dressings
- Part X: domiciliary oxygen therapy service
- Part XV: borderline substances
- Part XVI: notes on charges
- Part XVII A: dental prescribing
- Part XVII B: nurse and extended nurse prescribing
- Part XVIII A: black/banned list
- Part XVIII B: SLS list
- Index

styles 1–4 are given below, and Table 1.6 reviews the vocabulary used in MCQs and provides a guide to interpretation.

MCQ style 1: Simple completion type

These are set out as either incomplete statements or questions which require one answer from a choice of five answers. It is important to look carefully at the wording; phrasing the question negatively or using exceptions to a rule can alter the meaning of it. Read incomplete statements as a whole by inserting your answer in the missing space. If you have to guess the answer, try to eliminate as many choices as possible.

Table 1.6 Meanings of words and phrases used in questions

Words or phrases	Meaning
'must', 'should', 'could'	Questions with these words require some form of action to be taken. (You can substitute these words with 'have to' for ease of understanding.)
'best', 'appropriate', 'optimum'	These are 'red herrings', as there is only one correct option from the five choices
'over-the-counter' (OTC)	Medicinal products that do not require a prescription for purchase
'not', 'except'	Wording creates a negative question

Example of MCQ style 1: Simple completion type

Select the most appropriate answer for each of the following questions or incomplete statements.

Ampicillin should not be given for:
A: *exacerbation of chronic bronchitis*
B: *blind treatment of a sore throat*
C: *gonorrhoea*
D: *UTI*
E: *middle-ear infection*

Answer: B.

MCQ style 2: Classification type

Questions are grouped together, and the same five choices are used to select one answer for each question. These questions are very similar in style to the simple completion type (MCQ style 1). The answer to each question should not be influenced by the previous answer as it is possible for more than one question to have the same answer.

Example of MCQ style 2: Classification type

For each question select the appropriate lettered option. The letter options within a group of questions may be used once, more than once, or not used.

Questions (a) and (b) concern the following reference sources:
A: *Martindale: The Extra Pharmacopoeia*
B: *Drug Tariff*
C: *Medicines, Ethics and Practice: a Guide for Pharmacists*
D: *British National Formulary*
E: *British Pharmacopoeia*

Which one of the above is the correct answer to the following?

(a) *Contains the report form for suspected adverse drug reactions*
(b) *Provides a list of over-the-counter medicines liable to abuse*

(a) Answer: D.
(b) Answer: C.

MCQ style 3: Multiple completion type

Each question has three responses, of which one or more may be correct. The main difficulty of this style of question is to ensure that your answer reflects what you think is the correct combination of responses.

Example of MCQ style 3: Multiple completion type

Three responses accompany each question. Choose as your answer, from A to E, which of the following is appropriate:

A: *1, 2 and 3 are correct*
B: *1 and 2 correct only*
C: *2 and 3 correct only*
D: *1 correct only*
E: *3 correct only*

Summary of correct responses

A: 1, 2, 3	B: 1, 2 only	C: 2, 3 only	D: 1 only	E: 3 only

Which of the following is appropriate treatment for a nose bleed:

1 *sit patient down*
2 *tip the head back*
3 *apply pressure above the nasal bridge*

Answer: D.

MCQ style 4: Assertion–reason type

Each question consists of two statements, each of which requires a true or false answer. If you decide that both statements are true then the second statement has to be considered if it is the correct explanation of the first statement. The easiest approach to answering these questions is to insert the word 'because' between the two true statements and then determine, if taken together, they make sense.

Assertion–reason questions require a lot of thought, and care is needed to ensure that your answer reflects what you think is the correct response.

Example of MCQ style 4: Assertion–reason type

The following questions consist of two statements. Choose as your answer, from A to E, which of the following is appropriate.

A: *both statements are true and the second statement is a correct explanation of the first statement*
B: *both statements are true, but the second statement is not a correct explanation of the first statement*
C: *the first statement is true but the second statement is false*
D: *the first statement is false but the second statement is true*
E: *both statements are false*

Question:

1st statement: pseudoephedrine should not be given with phenelzine
2nd statement: phenelzine is an MAO-B inhibitor

Answer: C.

Summary of correct responses

1st statement	2nd statement	
A True	True	2nd statement is correct explanation of 1st statement
B True	True	2nd statement is not correct explanation of 1st statement
C True	False	
D False	True	
E False	False	

Problems before, during and after the exam

Figure 1.1 illustrates the options if you have difficulties either before or during the exam.

For most preregistration students, notification of the examination results will be 4–6 weeks before the end of their training period. Whether a candidate has been successful or not can be determined without opening the results letter: a small thin letter indicates a pass, whereas a large thick one does not.

For those unfortunate not to have passed, their results letter will summarise the topic areas which the exam has highlighted as being weak. Such candidates ought to, with their preregistration tutor, analyse and review the exam performance and training in order to address how these weaknesses may be overcome. For the remaining period of employment, a work schedule should be planned and followed so that the candidate may gain as much experience as possible to overcome his or her own weak areas of pharmacy practice. Additional assistance may be sought by learning from the experiences of other preregistration students.

An appeals process does exist. However, a failed candidate can request that their exam result be reconsidered only on the following grounds:

- the candidate believes that the examination procedures were not correctly followed, or

- further information, about the candidate's ability to perform the exam, has become available which could not be given prior to, or after, the fifth day of the examination.

It should be borne in mind that an appeal is unlikely to succeed if any information submitted with the application has already been seen by the examiners.

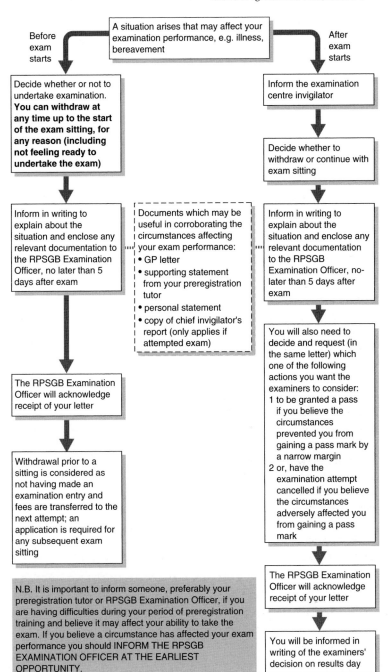

Figure 1.1 What to do if there are circumstances affecting an examination performance.

Closed book questions

STYLE 1 – SIMPLE COMPLETION TYPE

Select the most appropriate answer for each of the following questions or incomplete statements. (*For Answers, see Chapter 7.*)

2.1 Doxycycline should not be taken at the same time of day with medicines containing iron because:

    A: *the side-effects of doxycycline will be increased*
    B: *the side-effects of iron will be increased*
    C: *the excretion of iron is decreased*
    D: *the absorption of doxycycline may be decreased*
    E: *the metabolism of doxycycline may be increased*

2.2 Mrs W takes warfarin 5 mg daily to treat atrial fibrillation. At a recent clinic appointment her international normalised ratio (INR) was found to be 5. Which one of the following statements is correct?

    A: *phenindione should be taken instead of warfarin*
    B: *determine if Mrs W has recently increased her intake of green vegetables*
    C: *the warfarin dose should be increased*
    D: *the warfarin dose should be decreased*
    E: *the current dose of warfarin is appropriate*

2.3 Which one of the following body mass index values is an indication of obesity?

    A: *7*
    B: *15*
    C: *22*
    D: *28*
    E: *33*

2.4 Which of the following is a common side-effect of glyceryl trinitrate?

A: *constipation*
B: *flushing*
C: *fine tremor*
D: *sleep disturbance*
E: *vomiting*

2.5 Ms R suffers from acute migraine attacks. Her GP should prescribe:

A: *clonidine*
B: *methysergide*
C: *naratriptan*
D: *pizotifen*
E: *propranolol*

2.6 The following is written on a prescription:

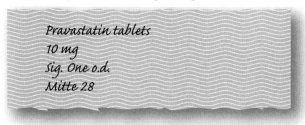

Pravastatin tablets
10 mg
Sig. One o.d.
Mitte 28

You should advise the patient to take this medication:

A: *in the morning*
B: *at lunchtime*
C: *mid-afternoon*
D: *at night*
E: *after a meal*

2.7 Which of the following is unlikely to cause nausea and/or vomiting during the initial stages of treatment?

A: *cardiac glycosides*
B: *non-steroidal anti-inflammatory drugs*
C: *oral contraceptives*
D: *phenothiazines*
E: *prostaglandin analogues*

2.8 Asthma patients should not take:

A: *atenolol*
B: *metronidazole*
C: *phenytoin*
D: *salbutamol*
E: *warfarin*

2.9 Mr K suffers from schizophrenia and does not regularly take his oral antipsychotic medication. His GP wants to switch him to intramuscular depot injections and asks for your advice about the appropriate dosing intervals. Your reply should be:

A: *daily*
B: *every 2 to 3 days*
C: *every 1 to 4 weeks*
D: *twice a year*
E: *annually*

2.10 You are the ward pharmacist and undertake a drug history of Mr T who was admitted to hospital as a result of a gastrointestinal haemorrhage. His medication on admission is:

- *Bendroflumethiazide tablets 2.5 mg every morning*
- *Fluoxetine capsules 20 mg daily*
- *Ketoprofen capsules 100 mg twice a day with food*
- *Propranolol tablets 80 mg twice a day*
- *Suscard® (glyceryl trinitrate) buccal tablets 1 mg three times daily*

The GI bleed may be attributed to which of the following drug regimes?

A: *Bendroflumethiazide*
B: *Fluoxetine*
C: *Ketoprofen*
D: *Propranolol*
E: *Suscard® (glyceryl trinitrate)*

2.11 A GP informs you that Mike B was unable to obtain dexamethasone oral solution, which is immediately required. Mike B is 9 years old and receives regular prescriptions for salbutamol and budesonide inhalers. Which of the following statements would be appropriate advice to give to the GP?

A: *increase the use of the budesonide inhaler*

B: *initiate additional prophylaxis for asthma using sodium cromoglicate inhaler at 10 mg four times daily*

C: *inform the GP when the oral solution will become available from the manufacturer*

D: *continue existing inhaler treatment and substitute prednisolone soluble tablets at an equivalent (dexamethasone) dose*

E: *continue existing inhaler treatment and use a reducing dose regime of prednisolone enteric-coated tablets*

2.12 The appearance of a generalised skin rash following a course of ampicillin treatment is suggestive of what condition?

A: *endocarditis*

B: *glandular fever*

C: *meningitis*

D: *renal insufficiency*

E: *urinary tract infection*

2.13 Which one of the following is a symptom of digoxin toxicity?

A: *decreased blood pressure*

B: *dry mouth*

C: *increased heart rate*

D: *skin rash*

E: *vomiting*

2.14 Caution should be applied to which one of the following drugs in a patient with migraine?

A: *amitriptyline*

B: *combined oral contraceptives*

C: *metoclopramide*

D: *sumatriptan*

E: *tolfenamic acid*

2.15 What is the main advantage of administering glyceryl trinitrate via the sublingual route?

A: *increased first-pass (hepatic) metabolism*
B: *rapid onset of action*
C: *reduced incidence of headache*
D: *reduced tolerance*
E: *short duration of action*

2.16 The presence of food in the stomach does not affect the oral absorption of which one of the following drugs?

A: *amoxicillin*
B: *ampicillin*
C: *flucloxacillin*
D: *phenoxymethylpenicillin*
E: *ketoconazole*

2.17 Which side-effect is not attributed to a tricyclic antidepressant?

A: *blurred vision*
B: *diarrhoea*
C: *sedation*
D: *sweating*
E: *urinary retention*

2.18 In order to prevent occurrence of neural tube defect women who are planning a pregnancy should be advised to take what following daily dose of folic acid?

A: *100 micrograms*
B: *200 micrograms*
C: *300 micrograms*
D: *400 micrograms*
E: *500 micrograms*

2.19 Thiazide diuretics are unlikely to cause which one of the following?

A: *onset of action is within 2 hours of oral administration*
B: *may cause hyperkalaemia*
C: *may cause hypokalaemia*
D: *may cause hypercalcaemia*
E: *may precipitate diabetes mellitus*

2.20 Preparations containing aluminium, calcium or magnesium salts can inhibit the gut absorption of which one of the following?

A: *cefalexin*
B: *chloramphenicol*
C: *erythromycin*
D: *phenoxymethylpenicillin*
E: *tetracycline*

2.21 Ms P hands you a prescription for the following:

> • *Isoniazid 300 mg daily*
> • *Rifampicin 600 mg daily*
> • *Cilest o.d.*

She should be advised to take additional contraceptive precautions due to:

A: *isoniazid reduces absorption of oestrogens and progestrogens*
B: *isoniazid increases oestrogen metabolism by the liver*
C: *rifampicin causes increased protein binding of progestrogens*
D: *rifampicin increases oestrogen and progestogen metabolism by the liver*
E: *rifampicin and isoniazid increase oestrogen metabolism by the liver*

2.22 With which one of the following are patients advised to use a wide-spectrum sunscreen?

A: *amiodarone*
B: *clopidogrel*
C: *digoxin*
D: *glyceryl trinitrate*
E: *sotalol*

2.23 Which of the following does not have a potential interaction with phenelzine?

A: *alcohol*
B: *mature cheese*
C: *fresh orange juice*
D: *well-hung game*
E: *yeast extract*

Section II

STYLE 2 – CLASSIFICATION TYPE

For each question select the appropriate lettered option. The letter options within a group of questions may be used once, more than once, or not used. (*For Answers, see Chapter 7.*)

Questions 2.24 to 2.28 relate to the following drugs:

A: *ciprofloxacin*
B: *ketoconazole*
C: *nystatin*
D: *rifampicin*
E: *tetracycline*

Which one of the above:

2.24 Induces hepatic enzyme activity *D*

2.25 May cause body secretions to be coloured orange-red *D*

2.26 May induce convulsions *A*

2.27 Does not result in systemic absorption when administered orally *C*

2.28 Chelates iron, calcium and magnesium ions in the gastrointestinal tract *E*

Question 2.29 to 2.31 concern the following:

A: *acarbose*
B: *gliclazide*
C: *glibenclamide*
D: *metformin*
E: *rosiglitazone*

Choose from A to E for the following statements:

2.29 Reduces peripheral insulin resistance *B*

2.30 Delays the digestion and absorption of starch and sucrose

A

2.31 Drug of first choice in overweight patients with diabetes mellitus *D*

Questions 2.32 to 2.34 concern the following medicines:

A: *bendroflumethiazide*
B: *clomethiazide*
C: *digoxin*
D: *fluphenazine*
E: *ramipril*

Which drug is associated with the following side-effect:

2.32 Hyperglycaemia *A*

2.33 Renal impairment *E*

2.34 Extrapyramidal symptoms *D*

Questions 2.35 and 2.36 concern the following drugs used in epilepsy:

A: *carbamazepine*
B: *ethosuximide*
C: *phenobarbital*
D: *phenytoin*
E: *sodium valproate*

Which one of the anti-epileptics displays the following characteristics:

2.35 Has non-linear pharmacokinetics

2.36 Concurrent administration with voriconazole may lead to increased effects of this drug

The following antibiotics relate to questions 2.37 to 2.39:

A: *amoxicillin 250 mg capsules*
B: *ciprofloxacin 250 mg tablets*
C: *erythromycin 250 mg tablets*
D: *oxytetracycline 250 mg tablets*
E: *vancomycin 125 mg capsules*

Select, from A to E, which one of the above:

2.37 Should be avoided in penicillin-allergic patients *A*

2.38 Is an alternative to penicillin in hypersensitive patients *C*

2.39 Is used to treat antibiotic-associated (pseudomembranous) *E*
colitis

Questions 2.40 and 2.41 concern the following drug doses:

    A: *atenolol 50 mg o.d.*
    B: *dosulepin 75 mg o.d.*
    C: *finasteride 5 mg o.m.*
    D: *methotrexate 7.5 mg o.d.*
    E: *quinidine 200 mg t.d.s.*

    Select, from A to E, which one of the above is:

2.40 An unlicensed indication in women *C*

2.41 An inappropriate dose *D*

Questions 2.42 to 2.44 relate to the following drugs:

    A: *amiodarone*
    B: *furosemide*
    C: *cholestyramine*
    D: *heparin*
    E: *levothyroxine*

    Select which of the above interferes with the effects of digoxin by:

2.42 Increasing digoxin plasma concentration *A*

2.43 Increasing the risk of digoxin toxicity as a result of
hypokalaemia *B*

2.44 Reducing digoxin absorption *C*

Section III

STYLE 3 – MULTIPLE COMPLETION TYPE

Three responses accompany each question. Choose as your answer, from A to E, which of the following is appropriate. (*For answers, see Chapter 7.*)

> A: *1, 2 and 3 are correct*
> B: *1 and 2 correct only*
> C: *2 and 3 correct only*
> D: *1 correct only*
> E: *3 correct only*

2.45 The effects of hormone replacement therapy (HRT) include:

E

1. *providing contraceptive cover*
2. *reducing the risk of developing breast cancer*
3. *reducing the risk of developing postmenopausal osteoporosis*

2.46 Which of the following has an indication for the treatment of gout?

A

1. *allopurinol*
2. *colchicine*
3. *diclofenac*

2.47 Which of the following are appropriate for the treatment of acute attacks of gout?

E

1. *aspirin*
2. *allopurinol*
3. *colchicine*

2.48 The brand should be specified when prescribing for which of the following preparations?

A

1. *carbamazepine tablets*
2. *lithium tablets*
3. *theophylline m/r tablets*

2.49 Additional contraceptive precautions should be used in the following therapies:

B

1. *carbamazepine*
2. *phenobarbital*
3. *rabeprazole*

2.50 Patients on warfarin tablets should be informed on the following:

1 inform their doctor if they experience bleeding or bruising problems
2 not take any analgesics unless advised by their doctor
3 not drink alcohol

2.51 Symptoms of lithium toxicity may present as:

1 increasing gastrointestinal disturbance
2 euphoria
3 photosensitivity

2.52 Alcohol should be avoided in which of the following drugs?

1 amitriptyline
2 disulfiram
3 ranitidine

2.53 Which of the following methods of drug delivery may be used to avoid hepatic first-pass metabolism?

1 metered dose inhaler
2 sublingual tablets
3 transdermal patches

2.54 Lipid-soluble drugs exhibit the following characteristics:

1 undergo renal excretion without being changed
2 penetrate the central nervous system
3 have a high apparent volume of distribution

2.55 Which of the following drugs will increase in the plasma concentration of theophylline?

1 diltiazem
2 fluconazole
3 tobacco

2.56 Asthmatics, who use theophylline as part of their treatment, should not take cimetidine because:

1 plasma concentrations of theophylline will be reduced
2 they may experience increased incidences of headache and nausea
3 the dose of theophylline may need to be altered

2.57 Patients with poor inhaler technique may be advised to use which of the following devices?

A

1 *a breath-actuated pressured inhaler*
2 *a dry powder inhaler*
3 *a space device with a metered-dose inhaler*

2.58 Which of the following are characteristics of large-volume intravenous infusions?

B

1 *be isotonic*
2 *be free from particles*
3 *be preservative-free*

2.59 The prescriber should be contacted in which of the following incidences?

B

1 *a prescription for atorvastatin and gemfibrozil*
2 *a prescription for misoprostol for a woman who is 23 weeks pregnant*
3 *a prescription for paracetamol for a 2-year-old child*

2.60 Ibuprofen:

A

1 *exhibits analgesic, anti-inflammatory and anti-pyretic properties*
2 *inhibits release of prostaglandin*
3 *has a peripheral analgesic action*

Section IV

STYLE 4 – ASSERTION–REASON TYPE

The following questions consist of two statements. Choose as your answer, from A to E, which of the following is appropriate. (*For Answers, see Chapter 7.*)

> A: both statements are true and the second statement is a correct explanation of the first statement
> B: both statements are true, but the second statement is not a correct explanation of the first statement
> C: the first statement is true but the second statement is false
> D: the first statement is false but the second statement is true
> E: both statements are false

2.61 **1st statement:** patients with severe liver disease should avoid taking warfarin

A

2nd statement: warfarin can cause hepatic encephalopathy

2.62 Mr S has been prescribed the following new medicines:

> Indapamide 2.5 mg o.m.
> Lithium 200 mg b.d.

D

1st statement: a potentially hazardous interaction may occur with this combination of drugs

2nd statement: sodium toxicity enhances lithium toxicity

2.63 Mrs J takes phenobarbital tablets 60 mg each night for partial seizures and has three tablets remaining. She has given her repeat prescription to her GP surgery but comes into your pharmacy asking for an emergency supply of phenobarbital, in case her doctor does not issue a new prescription in time.

B

1st statement: missed doses of phenobarbital can result in an epileptic seizure

2nd statement: rebound seizures may be a problem if phenobarbital is stopped

2.64 **1st statement:** administration of insulin should be via the intravenous or intramuscular route when treating patients with diabetic ketoacidosis

C

2nd statement: insulin absorption may be slow and erratic when administered from subcutaneous injection

2.65 **1st statement:** Septrin® (co-trimoxazole) should not be taken by women in the last trimester of pregnancy

B

2nd statement: sulphonamides are a folate antagonist

2.66 **1st statement:** patients with diabetes mellitus should decrease their insulin intake during periods of illness

A

2nd statement: there is a decrease in the demand for insulin when the body is under stress

2.67 **1st statement:** foods high in fat should be avoided for 14 days by patients undergoing treatment withdrawal of monoamine-oxidase inhibitors (MAOIs)

E

2nd statement: tyramine may increase the pressor effect of MAOIs for up to 14 days after treatment has stopped

2.68 **1st statement:** oral nystatin is not used for the treatment of vaginal candidiasis

A

2nd statement: nystatin is not absorbed from the gastrointestinal tract

2.69 **1st statement:** diuretic treatment should be briefly stopped
✓ prior to initiating an ACE inhibitor in a patient with congestive
heart failure

A **2nd statement:** ACE inhibitors can exacerbate hypokalaemia
induced by thiazide and loop diuretics

2.70 **1st statement:** patients on warfarin treatment should be
advised not to take aspirin
C **2nd statement:** aspirin can produce a gastrointestinal
haemorrhage

Open book questions

STYLE 1 – SIMPLE COMPLETION TYPE

Select the most appropriate answer for each of the following questions or incomplete statements. (*For Answers, see Chapter 7.*)

2.71 Which of the following would be a suitable daily dose for a 3-year-old child receiving trimethoprim for prophylaxis of recurrent urinary tract infections?

A: *2 mg*
B: *25 mg*
C: *30 mg*
D: *50 mg*
E: *100 mg*

2.72 Mr C regularly takes glibenclamide to control type 2 diabetes mellitus. Which one of the following drugs can have an undesired effect on Mr C's blood glucose levels?

A: *aspirin*
B: *atorvastatin*
C: *doxazosin*
D: *indapamide*
E: *tramadol*

2.73 Mrs K is a regular patient of your pharmacy. She takes one Tildiem LA® 200 mg capsule every morning and asks you if she is allowed to drink grapefruit juice with this medication. You advise her that:

A: *Tildiem LA® and grapefruit juice should be taken separately at least 2 hours apart*
B: *Tildiem LA® should be stopped and her blood pressure measured after 1 week*
C: *drink only long-life grapefruit juice, and not the fresh variety*
D: *grapefruit juice is not known to be hazardous when taking Tildiem LA®*
E: *to visit her GP and ask for an alternative to Tildiem LA®*

2.74 Which one of the following antibiotics is contraindicated in a patient with a glomerular filtration rate (GFR) of 35 ml/ minute?

A: *amoxicillin*
B: *cefalexin*
C: *ciprofloxacin*
D: *erythromycin*
E: *oxytetracycline*

2.75 Mrs W is about to undergo a dental procedure that requires general anaesthesia. Her medical history reveals that she has a prosthetic heart valve and an allergy to penicillin. What choice of antibiotic(s) would you advise for the prevention of endocarditis?

A: *amoxicillin*
B: *cefotaxime*
C: *vancomycin*
D: *amoxicillin and gentamicin*
E: *vancomycin and gentamicin*

2.76 A practice nurse telephones you about a Mr F, who is 44 years old and has recently had his blood pressure measured. His blood pressure was 150/90 mmHg and he is at very low risk of developing coronary heart disease within the next 10 years. The nurse would like your advice regarding Mr F's blood pressure. Which of the following responses should you give?

A: *he should be started on an ACE inhibitor*
B: *he should be started on a thiazide diuretic*
C: *he should have his blood pressure reassessed at 6-monthly intervals*
D: *he should be advised about lifestyle changes*
E: *he should be advised to do nothing*

Questions 2.77 to 2.79 concern Mr T who regularly takes theophylline for his asthma. He smokes 25 cigarettes per day and drinks approximately 11 units of alcohol per week.

2.77 Mr T's plasma theophylline concentration was measured at the asthma clinic. The optimum plasma theophylline concentration for Mr T is:

A: *1–5 mg/litre*
B: *5–10 mg/litre*
C: *10–20 mg/litre*
D: *30–40 mg/litre*
E: *50–100 mg/litre*

2.78 Which of the following would you expect to observe if Mr T's plasma theophylline concentration is above the optimum range?

A: *drowsiness*
B: *hyperkalaemia*
C: *hypoglycaemia*
D: *tachycardia*
E: *visual disturbances*

2.79 Which of the following may result in an increase in plasma theophylline concentration?

A: *starting phenobarbital*
B: *starting primidone*
C: *starting warfarin*
D: *reducing alcohol intake*
E: *stopping smoking*

2.80 Which of the following would be a suitable infusion fluid for AmBisome® infusion?

A: *glucose 5% with pH ≥ 4.2*
B: *Ringer's solution pH ≥ 5.5*
C: *sodium chloride 0.9%*
D: *sodium chloride and glucose intravenous infusion*
E: *water for injections*

2.81 An appropriate treatment for an acute migraine attack is:

A: *clonidine*
B: *methysergide*
C: *naratriptan*
D: *pizotifen*
E: *propranolol*

2.82 What is the maximum allowed number of Cafergot® suppositories that may be used in any one week?

A: *2*
B: *4*
C: *6*
D: *8*
E: *10*

2.83 Ms K develops a skin rash after beginning a course of ampicillin capsules. What condition might she be suffering from?

A: *endocarditis*
B: *glandular fever*
C: *meningitis*
D: *renal insufficiency*
E: *urinary tract infection*

2.84 Which of the following side-effects is not associated with the stated drug?

A: *anaemia with propranolol*
B: *anorexia with methotrexate*
C: *diarrhoea with amoxicillin*
D: *hepatotoxicity with pyrazinamide*
E: *pseudomembranous colitis with clindamycin*

2.85 A nurse comes into the pharmacy and asks for your advice. An elderly patient of hers has recently been prescribed phenytoin and appears to be in a state of confusion. The nurse wants to know if this could be a side-effect of starting phenytoin. Your advice should be:

A: *phenytoin is unlikely to be the cause of this situation*
B: *advise her to contact the doctor for further advice*
C: *advise her that the dose of phenytoin may be too high and a plasma concentration should be taken*
D: *advise her that the dose of phenytoin should be reduced*
E: *advise her that phenytoin should be stopped*

2.86 Which one of the following is not a side-effect associated with the use of Oxis®?

A: *constipation*
B: *fine muscle spasm*
C: *headache*
D: *nervous tension*
E: *tachycardia*

2.87 Which one of the following water levels would it be advisable for children to be supplemented with oral fluoride?

A: *900 nanograms fluoride per ml*
B: *0.1 g fluoride per litre*
C: *0.007% fluoride*
D: *0.2 micrograms fluoride per ml*
E: *5 parts fluoride per million*

2.88 Which of the following statements is correct in relation to the interaction between warfarin and dipyridamole?

A: *this combination should never be dispensed*
B: *this combination is useful in the treatment of venous thromboembolism*
C: *this combination is useful in the prevention of thrombus formation on prosthetic heart valves*
D: *this is not a potentially hazardous interaction*
E: *phenindione is the preferred anticoagulant to use with dipyridamole*

2.89 What is the sodium ion concentration in a sodium chloride 0.9% infusion solution?

A: *50 mmol/l*
B: *100 mmol/l*
C: *150 mmol/l*
D: *200 mmol/l*
E: *500 mmol/l*

2.90 Which one of the following is not correct, with regard to gout treatment?

A: *allopurinol is not indicated for the treatment of an acute attack of gout*
B: *aspirin may be used for an acute attack of gout*
C: *colchicine can cause diarrhoea*
D: *patients with moderate renal impairment should not use probenecid*
E: *thiazide diuretics may precipitate gout*

Section II   *15 questions*

For each question select the appropriate lettered option. The letter options within a group of questions may be used once, more than once, or not used. (*For Answers, see Chapter 7.*)

Questions 2.91 to 2.93 relate to the following scenario:

Mr X is 73 years old and has recently been diagnosed with type 2 diabetes mellitus. His doctor is considering using the following antidiabetic drugs:

A: *chlorpropamide*
B: *gliclazide*
C: *glipizide*
D: *metformin*
E: *tolbutamide*

Select, from A to E, which one of the above:

2.91 Is unlikely to result in weight gain

2.92 Is most likely to cause lactic acidosis

2.93 Is most likely to produce hypoglycaemia

Questions 2.94 to 2.96 concern the following diuretics:

A: *bendroflumethiazide*
B: *bumetanide*
C: *furosemide*
D: *triamterene*
E: *torasemide*

Which one of the above applies to each of the following statements:

2.94 Is suitable for patients with liver disease

2.95 Can cause hyperkalaemia

2.96 Inhibits sodium re-absorption at the beginning of the distal convoluted tubule

Questions 2.97 to 2.100 concern the following:

> A: *ciprofloxacin*
> B: *clindamycin*
> C: *flucloxacillin*
> D: *ketoconazole*
> E: *rifampicin*
>
> Which of the above antibiotics:

2.97 Should not be used in children

2.98 Has an indication for gonorrhoea

2.99 Discolours soft contact lenses

2.100 Should be discontinued if diarrhoea occurs

Questions 2.101 to 2.103 concern the following:

> A: *ampicillin*
> B: *ciprofloxacin*
> C: *gentamicin*
> D: *metronidazole*
> E: *nitrofurantoin*
>
> Which one of the above drugs do the following statements refer to?

2.101 Administration by the oral route is inappropriate as it is not sufficiently absorbed from the gut

2.102 Is recommended for treating *Campylobacter* enteritis infections

2.103 Is not recommended for a patient with a glomerular filtration rate of 40 ml/minute

Questions 2.104 and 2.105 concern the following beta-blockers:

> A: *bisoprolol*
> B: *celiprolol*
> C: *esmolol*
> D: *labetalol*
> E: *timolol*
>
> Select, from A to E, which one of the above drugs:

2.104 Can be used for prophylaxis after myocardial infarction (MI), if given in the early convalescent phase after an MI

2.105 Is used in the treatment of moderate or severe heart failure

Section III

STYLE 3 – MULTIPLE COMPLETION TYPE

Three responses accompany each question. Choose as your answer, from A to E, which of the following is appropriate. (*For Answers, see Chapter 7.*)

> A: *1, 2 and 3 are correct*
> B: *1 and 2 correct only*
> C: *2 and 3 correct only*
> D: *1 correct only*
> E: *3 correct only*

2.106 Women on Roaccutane® should be counselled to:

1 *take the medication with or after food*
2 *avoid wax epilation*
3 *use effective contraception*

2.107 Which of the following analgesics could be used in the first trimester of pregnancy?

1 *aspirin*
2 *ibuprofen*
3 *paracetamol*

2.108 Which of the following drugs do not require dose reductions in a patient with a glomerular filtration rate of 30 ml/minute?

1 *ampicillin*
2 *glimepiride*
3 *tamsulosin*

2.109 A child, 7 years of age, has been prescribed streptomycin injections as part of the treatment for tuberculosis. Which of the following statements is/are true?

1 *1 g is the required dose of streptomycin*
2 *hypercalcaemia may result from prolonged treatment*
3 *should be given by deep intramuscular injection*

2.110 Arrhythmias are a sign of overdose in which of the following drugs?

1 *perphenazine*
2 *diazepam*
3 *diclofenac*

2.111 Mr J is an asthmatic who regularly has the following medication:

> • *Budesonide 200 micrograms b.d.*
> • *Salbutamol 200 micrograms q.d.s p.r.n*
> • *Nuelin SA® 250 mg b.d.*

He is prescribed a course of antibiotics to treat a troublesome cough. Which of the following is/are unlikely to interact with his current medication?

1 amoxicillin
2 ciprofloxacin
3 erythromycin

2.112 Which of the following might be experienced if a patient were taking Coracten MR®?

1 blocked sinuses
2 constipation
3 urticaria

2.113 Which of the following are indications of a digoxin overdose?

1 dry mouth
2 fatigue
3 visual disturbances

2.114 Which of the following drugs may increase plasma theophylline concentration?

1 ciprofloxacin
2 diltiazem
3 fluvoxamine

2.115 Which of the following antibiotics is used in the treatment of *Campylobacter* enteritis?

1 ciprofloxacin
2 erythromycin
3 phenoxymethylpenicillin

2.116 Mr M is a patient on your hospital ward. You notice from his medical notes that he has a serum creatinine of less than 300 micromol/litre. Which of the following drugs should be avoided in his situation?

1 amoxicillin
2 gentamicin
3 nitrofurantoin

2.117 Which of the following statements applies to a paracetamol overdose?

1 methionine is an antidote to paracetamol poisoning
2 potentially lethal metabolites are produced
3 antidotes can only be given within 2 hours of ingesting paracetamol

2.118 Carbamazepine and sodium valproate may be used in combination to treat epilepsy. Which of the following statements are true?

1 there is a risk of blood dyscrasia
2 gingival hypertrophy may be a side-effect
3 long-term use of this combination is inadvisable

2.119 A patient with liver disease should avoid the following:

1 atorvastatin
2 entacapone
3 miconazole

2.120 Formoterol is a select beta$_2$-agonist used in the treatment of asthma. Other drugs in the same class include:

1 dobutamine
2 salbutamol
3 terbutaline

2.121 Which of the following are potentially hazardous interactions?

1 amiodarone and propranolol
2 amitriptyline and phenytoin
3 enalapril and lithium

2.122 Which of the following products can bring about acne?

  1 phenytoin
  2 progesterone
  3 topical corticosteroids

Section IV

STYLE 4 – ASSERTION–REASON TYPE

The following questions consist of two statements. Choose as your answer, from A to E, which of the following is appropriate. (*For Answers, see Chapter 7.*)

> A: *both statements are true and the second statement is a correct explanation of the first statement*
> B: *both statements are true, but the second statement is not a correct explanation of the first statement*
> C: *the first statement is true but the second statement is false*
> D: *the first statement is false but the second statement is true*
> E: *both statements are false*

2.123 **1st statement:** bumetanide is contraindicated in patients with congested cardiac failure receiving digoxin therapy

2nd statement: the risk of digoxin toxicity increases should hypokalaemia occur

Questions 2.124 and 2.125 concern a patient with staphylococcal endocarditis, which is to be treated with intravenous gentamicin and flucloxacillin.

2.124 **1st statement:** pre-dose and 1 hour post-dose blood samples should be taken to determine serum gentamicin concentrations

2nd statement: an effective serum gentamicin concentration for treating staphylococcal endocarditis is for the 1 hour post-dose to be 3–5 mg/litre and pre-dose to be less than 1 mg/litre

2.125 **1st statement:** the dose interval of gentamicin needs to be increased if the pre-dose serum concentration is above the recommended range

2nd statement: there is an increased risk of kidney impairment if gentamicin accumulates in the body

Questions 2.126 and 2.127 relate to the following drug history:

> *Alfacalcidol 1 microgram o.d.*
> *Furosemide 40 mg o.d.*
> *Gliquidone 60 mg t.d.s.*
> *Lisinopril 2.5 mg o.d.*
> *Phosex® one tablet b.d.*

2.126 **1st statement:** gliquidone should not be used in this patient

2nd statement: this patient has renal impairment

2.127 **1st statement:** enalapril should not be prescribed in this patient

2nd statement: glucose tolerance may be impaired by enalapril

Question 2.128 concerns an extract from a prescription:

> *Amoxicillin 250 mg q.d.s., mitte 1 OP*
> *Fluconazole 50 mg o.d., mitte 1 OP*
> *Glibenclamide 5 mg o.d., mitte 1 OP*

2.128 **1st statement:** there is a risk of hypoglycaemia occurring in this patient

2nd statement: amoxicillin increases the effect of glibenclamide

Question 2.129 relates to the following drug chart:

> Bendroflumethiazide 2.5 mg o.m.
> Digoxin 500 micrograms o.d.
> Tensipine MR ®40 mg b.d.
> Temazepam 10 mg o.n.

2.129 **1st statement:** the patient is at risk of digoxin toxicity

2nd statement: the dose of Tensipine MR® is inappropriate

2.130 **1st statement:** crystal violet paint may be purchased as an OTC product for the treatment of mouth ulcers

2nd statement: crystal violet paint has a licensed indication to be used on mucous membranes

Question 2.131 concerns counselling on the use of the oral progestogen-only contraceptive

2.131 **1st statement:** oral progestogen-only contraceptives are to be taken at the same time each day

2nd statement: contraceptive protection may be lost if plasma progestogen levels vary

2.132 **1st statement:** preparations containing paracetamol or paracetamol alone should not be taken when Solpadol® is used regularly

2nd statement: the maximum daily dose of paracetamol is 8 g

3   *Pharmacy Practice*

Pharmacy encompasses many topics, and the practising pharmacist would be expected to be aware of a wide range of issues, not just clinical drug use. Recent developments include continuing professional development; National Institute for Clinical Excellence (NICE) guidance on specific disease conditions and types of patients; and innovations in pharmacy practice.

Much of the information can be gained from the *Pharmaceutical Journal* (the official RPSGB publication for UK pharmacists) which all preregistration students should review on a regular basis. A general awareness of all issues affecting pharmacy is required for the purposes of the exam.

Tables 3.1–3.9 and Figure 3.1 summarise information that preregistration candidates would be expected to know, and may be examined in the actual exam. Practice questions follow the summaries.

Calendar packs and special containers

Special containers are used when the medication is effervescent or hygroscopic or when it is not practicable to dispense the exact prescribed quantity. Manufacturers' calendar packs are medicines in

Table 3.1 Pharmacy practice topics which may be examined

- Guidance and protocols for treating specific disease and patient groups
- NHS pharmaceutical services (e.g. professional fees, types of services offered)
- Innovations in pharmaceutical practice
- Continuing professional development (CPD)
- Communication skills
- Good pharmacy practice
- Good clinical practice
- Other healthcare services (e.g. NHS Direct, NHS walk-in centres)
- Clinical governance
- Principles of risk management

Table 3.2 Examples of clinical governance

Clinical governance principles	Examples
1. Quality improvement in the provision of services	• Written protocols and procedures • Staff training
2. Evidence-based practice	• Application of information derived from journals and current best practice
3. Risk-reduction strategies	• Use of PMRs for drug interactions • Appropriate questioning of customers to rule out serious illness (e.g. WWHAM)
4. CPD	• CPPE workshops and distance-learning packages • Clinical diplomas • Multidisciplinary CPD meetings
5. Informing good practice, ideas and innovation	• Newsletters • Staff and departmental meetings • CPPE meetings
6. Identifying poor performance	• RPSGB Inspectorate
7. Patient feedback	• Complaints procedure
8. Data collection systems	• EPOS data of OTC sales • PACT data

Table 3.3 Examples of special container items and calendar packs

Product	Original pack	Sub-pack
Alendronic acid tablets 70 mg[i]	4	–
Alfacalcidol capsules 0.25 mcg, 0.5 mcg and 1.0 mcg[i]	30	10
Cabergoline tablets 1 mg and 2 mg[i]	20	–
Cimetidine tablets 400 mg[♦]	60	15
Cimetidine tablets 800 mg[♦]	30	15
Co-triamterzide tablets 50/25[♦]	30	15
Dipyridamole m/r capsules 200 mg[i]	60	–
Fluoxetine hydrochloride capsules 20 mg[♦]	30	15
Glyceryl trinitrate tablets 300 mcg, 500 mcg and 600 mcg[i]	100	–
Nicorandil tablets 10 mg and 20 mg[i]	60	10
Oestrogens, conjugated tablets 625 mcg and 1.25 mg[♦]	84	28
Potassium chloride effervescent tablets 470 mg (potassium ions)[i]	20	20
Risedronate sodium tablets 5 mg and 30 mg[♦]	28	4

[i] Special containers.

[♦] Manufacturers' calendar packs.

Table 3.4 CRM guidelines on handling cytotoxic drugs

1. Cytotoxics should be reconstituted only by trained personnel
2. Designated areas should be assigned for the purpose of reconstituting cytotoxics
3. Protective clothing should be worn, including gloves and eye protection
4. Pregnant staff should not handle cytotoxics
5. Care is required to ensure safe disposal of waste material

Table 3.5 Treatment cards

Printed instructions should be given to patients on the following drugs:
- Anticoagulants
- Lithium
- Oral corticosteroids

Table 3.6 Storage temperatures

Phrase or term	Temperature
'Cold storage' or 'Refrigerator'	2–8°C
'Cool storage' or 'Store in cool place'	8–15°C
'Controlled room temperature'	Do not store above 25°C

Table 3.7 Categories of evidence[1]

1a: Evidence from meta-analysis of randomised controlled trials
1b: Evidence from at least one randomised controlled trial

2a: Evidence from at least one controlled study without randomisation
2b: Evidence from at least one other type of quasi-experimental study

3: Evidence from descriptive studies, e.g. comparative studies, correlations studies and case–control studies

4: Evidence from expert committee reports or opinions or clinical experience of respected authorities, or both

[1]Adapted from: Harbour R, Miller J A new system for grading recommendations in evidence based guidelines. *British Medical Journal* 2001; 323: 334–336.

Table 3.8 Strength of recommendation based on categories of evidence[1]

A: Directly based on category 1 evidence

B: Directly based on category 2 or extrapolated recommendation from category 1 evidence

C: Directly based on category 3 evidence or extrapolated recommendation from category 1 or 2 evidence

D: Directly based on category 4 evidence or extrapolated recommendation from category 1, 2 or 3 evidence

[1]Adapted from: Harbour R, Miller J. A new system for grading recommendations in evidence based guidelines. *British Medical Journal* 2001; 323: 334–336.

Table 3.9 Health-related organisations

Organisation	Functions
National Institute for Clinical Excellence (NICE)	• Tasked to appraise health techniques and produce clinical guidelines and best practice standards for the NHS in England and Wales • Appraise and issue guidance on clinical effectiveness and cost-effectiveness of drugs, technologies and treatments • Aims to ensure that all patients throughout England and Wales receive equitable treatment • http://www.nice.org.uk
National Service Frameworks (NSFs)	• Published national standards of care and interventions for a specified service or care group • Developed through an external reference group (ERG), i.e. health professionals, service users, carers, and other advocates • One NSF is expected to be published annually • http://www.publications.doh.gov.uk/nsf
National Electronic Library for Health (NeLH)	• Provides access to best current knowledge; and helps to improve health and health care clinical practice and patient choice • http://www.nelh.nhs.uk
The Cochrane Collaboration	• Prepares, maintains and disseminates systematic reviews of the effects of health care • http://www.cochrane.org

which the unit doses are packaged in blisters or strips showing the days of the week or month.

For items designated in the Drug Tariff as special containers, the pharmacist should dispense in the special container(s) the quantity nearest to that prescribed. In the case of calendar packs, the pharmacist can dispense the exact quantity prescribed, or packs or sub-packs nearest to the quantity prescribed. Reimbursement is determined by the quantity dispensed, and not on the prescribed quantity.

NHS Direct

NHS Direct is a nurse-led telephone and internet service for healthcare. It provides information about specific health queries, general information about health problems, and information about health services. Pharmacists are expected to be aware of the services provided by NHS Direct, and as such, questions may be (and indeed have been) set to examine this aspect of knowledge of preregistration pharmacists.

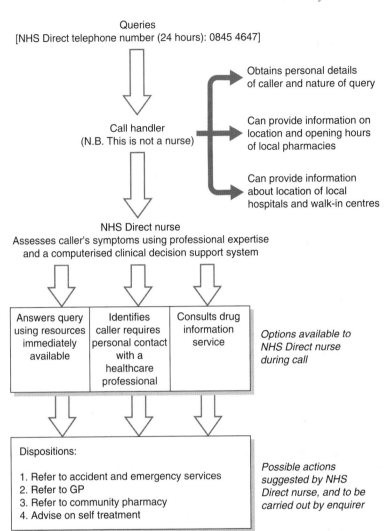

Figure 3.1 Summary of how enquiries to NHS Direct are resolved.

Section I

STYLE 1 – SIMPLE COMPLETION TYPE

Select the most appropriate answer for each of the following questions or incomplete statements. (*For Answers, see Chapter 7.*)

3.1 The best level of evidence to support the use of a particular therapy is:

A: *evidence from a systematic review of multiple, randomised, controlled trials*
B: *evidence from cohort studies*
C: *evidence from a randomised, controlled trial*
D: *evidence from non-experimental studies from more than one research group*
E: *expert opinion*

3.2 Pharmacists should carry out which one of the following statements when reporting adverse drug reactions to the Committee on Safety of Medicines?

A: *only report adverse reactions to any medicine with the inverted black triangle symbol ▼ in the BNF*
B: *only report severe adverse reactions to any medicine with the inverted black triangle symbol ▼ in the BNF*
C: *only report serious reactions to established medicines and all adverse reactions for medicines with the inverted black triangle symbol ▼ in the BNF*
D: *report adverse reactions to any medicine, unless the reaction is listed in the BNF*
E: *report all adverse reactions for medicines with the inverted black triangle symbol ▼ and serious reactions to established medicines, unless the reaction is listed in the BNF*

3.3 Concentrated chloroform water BP consists of 1 part
of chloroform diluted to 10 parts with aqueous diluent.
Chloroform water BP may be produced by diluting
concentrated chloroform water BP in which one of the
following proportions?

A: *concentrated chloroform water BP diluted 1 in 4 aqueous
diluent*

B: *concentrated chloroform water BP diluted 1 in 8 aqueous
diluent*

C: *concentrated chloroform water BP diluted 1 in 10 aqueous
diluent*

D: *concentrated chloroform water BP diluted 1 in 20 aqueous
diluent*

E: *concentrated chloroform water BP diluted 1 in 40 aqueous
diluent*

3.4 Clinical governance involves which one of the following?

A: *ensuring that patients receive appropriate and immediate
care*

B: *ensuring that resources are not wasted by NHS trusts*

C: *increasing investment of health promotion*

D: *improving the quality of services and safeguarding high
standards of care*

E: *improving the working conditions of NHS staff*

3.5 Which of the following is correct about an audit?

A: *is a component of quality assurance*

B: *must only be conducted in a community pharmacy*

C: *must implement the use of a patient survey*

D: *should only be conducted once on a particular topic*

E: *all pharmacists must conduct at least one audit per year*

3.6 How should glyceryl trinitrate tablets be dispensed?

A: *in glass containers with a child-resistant closure*

B: *in glass containers with a foil-lined cap containing cotton
wool wadding*

C: *in glass containers with a foil-lined cap containing no
cotton wool wadding*

D: *in plastic containers with a child-resistant closure and
cotton wool wadding*

E: *in plastic containers with a child-resistant closure and no
cotton wool wadding*

3.7 The main cause of aspirin degradation is:

A: *hydrolysis*
B: *oxidation*
C: *pH changes*
D: *photolysis*
E: *temperature*

3.8 The action of preservatives in pharmaceutical products is to:

A: *achieve sterility*
B: *eliminate microbial contamination during production*
C: *eliminate microbial contamination during use*
D: *eliminate pyrogens*
E: *satisfy regulatory requirements*

3.9 Which one of the following should a patient not do when using a beclometasone metered dose inhaler?

A: *carry a steroid warning card*
B: *after inhaling, hold the breath for 10 seconds*
C: *rinse the mouth with water after inhaling*
D: *shake the inhaler prior to use*
E: *use only when required*

3.10 Which one of the following is an unlikely explanation for the ineffectiveness of glyceryl trinitrate tablets?

A: *the patient suffers from a dry mouth*
B: *the patient has difficulty swallowing*
C: *the patient has developed tolerance to the effects of the drug*
D: *the drug has passed its expiry date*
E: *incorrect storage of the drug*

3.11 What is the temperature range for products to be stored in a refrigerator?

A: *−5–0°C*
B: *0–2°C*
C: *2–5°C*
D: *2–8°C*
E: *10–15°C*

3.12 It is a requirement for a pharmacist to endorse which one of the following on an NHS prescription, when dispensing a Schedule 2 or 3 controlled drug?

A: *CD*
B: *date of supply*
C: *manufacturer of dispensed product*
D: *quantity supplied*
E: *pack size*

3.13 Which one of the following is not a purpose of the Medicines and Healthcare products Regulatory Agency?

A: *assess applications for marketing authorisation*
B: *inspect drug production facilities*
C: *involved in drug recalls*
D: *monitoring compliance controlled drugs legislation*
E: *monitoring adverse drug reactions*

3.14 The recommended shelf-life of opened eye-drops in domiciliary use is:

A: *7 days*
B: *10 days*
C: *14 days*
D: *28 days*
E: *6 months*

3.15 Products labelled with 'store in a cool place' should not be stored in conditions exceeding which one of the following temperatures?

A: *5°C*
B: *10°C*
C: *15°C*
D: *20°C*
E: *25°C*

3.16 An NHS prescription for the following item is handed to you:

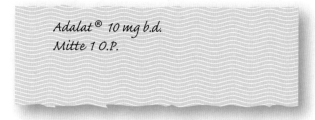

Adalat® 10 mg b.d.
Mitte 1 O.P.

You notice on the pharmacy PMR that the patient usually receives Adalat Retard® 10 mg tablets. Which one of the following actions should you take?

A: *contact the prescriber to clarify their intentions*
B: *dispense Adalat 10 mg capsules and endorse as such*
C: *dispense Adalat Retard 10 mg tablets and endorse as such*
D: *dispense Adalat Retard 10 mg tablets and return the prescription to the medical practitioner for endorsement*
E: *dispense nifedipine 10 mg capsules and endorse as such*

3.17 What is the shelf-life of an opened container of glyceryl trinitrate sublingual tablets?

A: *7 days*
B: *10 days*
C: *2 weeks*
D: *4 weeks*
E: *8 weeks*

Section II   *9 questions*

For each question select the appropriate lettered option. The letter options within a group of questions may be used once, more than once, or not used. (*For Answers, see Chapter 7.*)

Questions 3.18 to 3.24 concern the following:

A: *British National Formulary*
B: *Drug Tariff*
C: *Labelling on the packaging of commercially produced medicines*
D: *Martindale*
E: *Medicines, Ethics and Practice a Guide for Pharmacists*

Which one of the above would be an appropriate source of information for the following situations?

3.18 Determining the legal status of a medicinal product   E

3.19 Storage of controlled drugs as required by UK legislation E

3.20 Contact telephone numbers for drug information services A

3.21 Whether a medicinal product may be sold within the UK A

3.22 A report form for suspected adverse drug reactions A

3.23 Determining payment for maintaining patient records B

3.24 Ascertaining the number of NHS prescription charges for a particular medicinal product B

Questions 3.25 and 3.26 relate to the following cautionary labels for dispensed medicines:

A: *dissolve or mix with water before taking*

B: *do not stop taking this medicine except on your doctor's advice*

C: *do not take indigestion remedies at the same time as this medicine*

D: *warning: avoid alcoholic drink*

E: *warning: may cause drowsiness*

Select, from A to E, which cautionary label should be applied when dispensing the following medicines:

3.25 Metronidazole D

3.26 Rifampicin C

Section III   *19 questions*

Three responses accompany each question. Choose as your answer, from A to E, which of the following is appropriate. (*For Answers, see Chapter 7.*)

> A: *1, 2 and 3 are correct*
> B: *1 and 2 correct only*
> C: *2 and 3 correct only*
> D: *1 correct only*
> E: *3 correct only*

3.27 Which of the following should be undertaken prior to conducting an audit of prophylactic antibiotic use on a hospital surgical ward?

ß

1 *liaise with medical staff on the ward*
2 *obtain approval from the ethics committee*
3 *register any data obtained with the Data Protection Commissioner*

3.28 National Service Frameworks aim to do which of the following?

A

1 *establish national standards for clinical care*
2 *implement risk management strategies*
3 *reduce NHS costs*

3.29 Patients on glyceryl trinitrate sublingual tablets should be counselled to do which of the following?

C

1 *allowed a maximum of eight tablets within 24 hours*
2 *not to use any tablets after 8 weeks from opening the container*
3 *to place the tablet under the tongue and avoid swallowing*

3.30 You are presented with the following prescription:

> *Timolol eye drops 0.25% b.d.*
> *Theophylline m/r 250 mg b.d.*

Why should the prescriber be contacted?

1 *beta-blockers eye drops may not be appropriate for this patient, unless there is no suitable alternative available*
2 *the brand of theophylline should be specified* ✓
3 *theophylline plasma concentrations may increase as a result of systemic absorption of timolol eye-drops* ✓

3.31 Which of the following are examples of poor clinical governance?

1 *dispensing a non-repeatable prescription 10 months from the date of issue*
2 *incorrect dispensing of a prescription* ✓
3 *dispensing Oramorph® concentrated oral solution without an entry being made in the controlled drugs register*

3.32 An NHS prescription has been issued for Flagyl® (metronidazole) tablets. You have only generic metronidazole 200 mg tablets in stock. What action(s) could you take?

1 *dispense generic metronidazole 200 mg tablets and endorse as such*
2 *order Flagyl tablets and inform the patient when they can collect them*
3 *request a generically written prescription from the prescriber*

3.33 Which of the following are functions of the National Institute for Clinical Excellence?

1 *developing clinical guidelines*
2 *inspecting and monitoring the performance of NHS organisations*
3 *reducing health inequalities*

3.34 Which of the following should you do if a prescription has been incorrectly dispensed?

1 *apologise to the patient for the error and correctly dispense the prescription*
2 *determine how the error occurred and implement procedures to prevent it from happening again*
3 *inform the patient that you are personally not to blame, but it was another member of staff who made the error*

3.35 Pharmacists should be aware of which of the following?

1 *newly licensed medicines*
2 *new technologies affecting the practice of pharmacy*
3 *new health policies*

3.36 An audit provides a means to:

1 *determine the level of staff performance*
2 *identify and develop new areas of practice*
3 *improve standards of service*

3.37 Appropriate source(s) for obtaining drug information is/are:

1 *British National Formulary*
2 *hospital or manufacturers' drug information departments*
3 *a colleague using the same drug*

3.38 The storage of preserved liquid multiple-phase formulations in plastic containers may result in which of the following?

1 *decreased physical stability*
2 *microbial spoilage*
3 *reduction in drug content*

3.39 Which of the following statements applies to a newly licensed medicine?

1 *can be prescribed only by consultant physicians*
2 *doctors can only report suspected adverse reactions which may be attributed to the use of this medicine*
3 *the data sheet for the product would exhibit the inverted black triangle symbol* ▼

3.40 Suspected adverse reaction report forms should be submitted for which of the following?

1 *a blood dyscrasia following the use of an established drug*
2 *a severe skin eruption following administration of a vaccine*
3 *the development of a rash following treatment with a new antifungal*

3.41 Grade A (I) aseptic preparation areas require which of the following attributes?

1 *fresh sterile protective garments should be worn*
2 *the use of face masks to prevent the shedding of droplets*
3 *the provision of sinks and drains in aseptic areas*

3.42 Insulin preparations for injection should be:

1 *free from particles*
2 *stored at temperatures not above 0°C*
3 *sterile and pyrogen-free*

3.43 Devices for assisting patients with poor inhaler technique include:

1 *a breath-actuated powder inhaler*
2 *a collapsible extended mouthpiece with a metered dose inhaler*
3 *a spacer device with a metered dose inhaler*

3.44 How should the adsorbed diphtheria, tetanus, and [whole-cell] pertussis vaccine be stored?

1 *not be frozen*
2 *protected from light*
3 *stored at 2–8°C*

3.45 In order to ensure the quality of medicines, pharmacists should adopt which of the following practices?

1 *assign unique batch numbers to each batch of manufactured medicinal product*
2 *ensure that Good Manufacturing and Good Laboratory practices are adhered to before releasing a batch of medicinal product*
3 *be satisfied that the source of medicines is reputable*

STYLE 4 – ASSERTION–REASON TYPE

The following questions consist of two statements. Choose as your answer, from A to E, which of the following is appropriate. (*For Answers, see Chapter 7.*)

> A: *both statements are true and the second statement is a correct explanation of the first statement*
> B: *both statements are true, but the second statement is not a correct explanation of the first statement*
> C: *the first statement is true but the second statement is false*
> D: *the first statement is false but the second statement is true*
> E: *both statements are false*

3.46 **1st statement:** medicines returned by a patient, to a community pharmacy, should be examined for evidence of use or tampering before placing into stock

2nd statement: a pharmacist must be satisfied with the quality of medicines when fulfilling a prescription

3.47 **1st statement:** evidence-based information may be obtained from the Cochrane Library

2nd statement: the functions of the Cochrane Collaboration are to prepare, maintain and promote the accessibility of systematic reviews concerning the effects of healthcare interventions

3.48 **1st statement:** the Consumer Protection Act 1987 states that sole liability remains with the pharmacist when repackaging items into smaller quantities from bulk packs

2nd statement: the pharmacist should ensure that the label of the smaller pack has information that allows identification of the manufacturer and the batch of the bulk pack

3.49 **1st statement:** the dispensing label for metronidazole should contain a warning to avoid alcohol

2nd statement: alcohol delays the absorption of metronidazole from the gut

3.50 **1st statement:** the preferred method of sterilisation of aqueous preparations is by heating in an autoclave at a minimum temperature of 121°C for 15 minutes

2nd statement: heat sterilisation is the method of choice if it remains possible

3.51 **1st statement:** many vaccines require refrigeration as part of the ideal storage conditions

2nd statement: vaccines may become denatured and ineffective if not stored within the recommended temperature range

3.52 **1st statement:** oil-based preparations should not come into contact with contraceptive diaphragms or condoms

2nd statement: the latex rubber material of condoms and contraceptive diaphragms may be damaged by oil-based preparations

Open book questions

STYLE 1 – SIMPLE COMPLETION TYPE

Select the most appropriate answer for each of the following questions or incomplete statements. (*For Answers, see Chapter 7.*)

3.53 You are presented with the following items on an NHS prescription:

> *Prempak-C 0.625, 1 O.P.*
> *Scholl Class II thigh stocking, 1 pair*
> *Zoton 15 mg, 2 O.P.*

How many prescription charges are there for this prescription, if the patient is not exempt from payment?

A: 0
B: 1
C: 3
D: 4
E: 5

3.54 Analog XP® may only be allowed on an NHS prescription for which of the following conditions?

A: *patients with calcium intolerance*
B: *patients with glycogen storage disease*
C: *patients with long-chain acyl-CoA dehydrogenase deficiency*
D: *patients with phenylketonuria*
E: *patients with Refsum's disease*

3.55 An NHS prescription for Voltarol tablets 50 mg and Voltarol Retard tablets 100 mg is presented at your pharmacy. If the patient is not exempt from prescription payment, how many charges should you make?

A: 0

B: 1

C: 2

D: 3

E: 4

3.56 Which one of the following would require a report to be made for all suspected adverse reactions?

A: Carylderm®

B: Ecostatin®

C: Lescol®

D: Strefen®

E: Zibor®

3.57 The Advisory Committee on Borderline Substances has approved which one of the following to be prescribed on an FP10 prescription for a patient with renal failure?

A: Enlive® liquid

B: Enrich® liquid

C: Maxijul® liquid

D: MSUD Aid III® powder

E: Nepro® liquid

3.58 Which one of the following items carries only one prescription charge?

A: Climagest tablets

B: Estracombi TTS

C: Germoloids complete

D: Hypovase BD starter pack

E: Trisequens

3.59 Which one of the following is correct in relation to reporting suspected adverse reactions to the Medicines and Healthcare products Regulatory Agency?

A: *all suspected adverse drug reactions in children should be reported*

B: *the inverted black triangle symbol ▼ is used to identify medicines liable to produce adverse reactions*

C: *doctors should only initiate reporting of adverse reactions*

D: *minor adverse reactions resulting from newly licensed medicines should not be reported*

E: *suspected adverse reactions resulting from herbal products should not be reported*

3.60 Which one of the following would be passed for payment by the Prescription Pricing Authority if prescribed on an NHS prescription?

A: *Aproten® biscuits*

B: *OptiPen Pro®*

C: *Uristix® strips*

D: *Valium® tablets 2 mg*

E: *Xanax® tablets 500 micrograms*

3.61 The age that children are routinely vaccinated against rubella is:

A: *2 months*

B: *12–15 months*

C: *2 years*

D: *4–5 years*

E: *10–14 years*

3.62 Which one of the following is not exempt from NHS prescription charges?

A: *prescription of 30 tablets of norethisterone 5 mg for a 25-year-old woman*

B: *prescription for Galfer FA® for a pregnant woman of 25 weeks*

C: *prescription for Femulen® tablets for a 30-year-old woman*

D: *prescription for 100 co-proxamol tablets for a 40-year-old man with type 1 diabetes mellitus*

E: *prescription for salbutamol 100 microgram inhalers for a 67-year-old man*

3.63 Which one of the following may be kept in a monitored dosage system?

A: *GTN 300 mcg*
B: *Kloref® tablets*
C: *Losec MUPS® 10 mg*
D: *methotrexate 2.5 mg tablets*
E: *prednisolone 5 mg e/c tablets*

3.64 Which of the following situations would require two payable charges if you were presented with an NHS prescription?

A: *a 32-year-old woman prescribed Microgynon 30® tablets and diclofenac 50 mg tablets*
B: *a pregnant woman of 19 weeks prescribed Ferrogard Folic® tablets and paracetamol tablets*
C: *a 28-year-old woman prescribed Canesten Combi® and zopiclone 3.75 mg tablets*
D: *a 58-year-old woman prescribed one pair of Class II thigh-length stockings*
E: *a 68-year-old woman with diabetes mellitus prescribed metformin 500 mg tablets and Clinistix®*

3.65 What proportion of emulsifying wax is contained in aqueous cream?

A: *6% w/w*
B: *9% w/w*
C: *12% w/w*
D: *15% w/w*
E: *30% w/w*

Section II   *11 questions*

For each question select the appropriate lettered option. The letter options within a group of questions may be used once, more than once, or not used. (*For Answers, see Chapter 7.*)

Questions 3.66 to 3.71 concern the following number of prescription charges:

A: *0 charges*
B: *1 charge*
C: *2 charges*
D: *3 charges*
E: *4 charges*

Select, from A to E, the number of charges required for the following NHS prescriptions:

3.66 An epileptic with a prescription for gabapentin 100 mg capsules and gabapentin 600 mg tablets

3.67 A 25-year-old with a prescription for chlordiazepoxide 5 mg capsules and chlordiazepoxide 5 mg tablets

3.68 A 55-year-old man with a prescription for propranolol 10 mg tablets and propranolol 40 mg tablets

3.69 A 26-year-old man with a prescription for ibuprofen 200 mg tablets and ibuprofen 800 mg m/r tablets

3.70 A 47-year-old woman with a prescription for two packs of Micropore® tape 1.25 cm × 5 m and two packs of Micropore® tape 2.5 cm × 5 m

3.71 A 34-year-old woman with a prescription for Gynol II® and applicator

Questions 3.72 and 3.73 relate to the following antibiotics:

    A: *cefradine 250 mg capsules*
    B: *doxycycline 100 mg capsules*
    C: *fluconazole 50 mg capsules*
    D: *metronidazole 400 mg tablets*
    E: *minocycline 50 mg tablets*

    Which one of the above applies to the following statements:

3.72 Has an indication for giardiasis

3.73 Is not passed for payment by the Prescription Pricing Authority if issued on an NHS dental prescription

Questions 3.74 to 3.76 concern the following topical preparations:

    A: *Alphaderm® cream*
    B: *Betnovate-C® ointment*
    C: *Betnovate-RD® cream*
    D: *Halciderm Topical® cream*
    E: *Synalar N® cream*

    Select, from A to E, which of one of the preparations:

3.74 Is able to stain clothing

3.75 Is a 'very potent' topical corticosteroid

3.76 Contains hydroxybenzoates

Three responses accompany each question. Choose as your answer, from A to E, which of the following is appropriate. (*For Answers, see Chapter 7.*)

> A: *1, 2 and 3 are correct*
> B: *1 and 2 correct only*
> C: *2 and 3 correct only*
> D: *1 correct only*
> E: *3 correct only*

3.77 It would be appropriate to inform the Medicines and Healthcare products Regulatory Agency regarding the occurrence of adverse effects in which of the following products?

> 1 *contact lens fluids*
> 2 *dental materials*
> 3 *X-ray contrast media*

3.78 Which of the following statements concern cabergoline tablets?

> 1 *to be dispensed in the original container*
> 2 *have a shelf-life of 28 days after first opening the container*
> 3 *should be dissolved under the tongue*

3.79 Which of the following would require the prescribing of an alternative preparation if initially prescribed on an NHS dental prescription?

> 1 *benzydamine mouthwash 0.15%*
> 2 *isotretinoin gel 0.05%*
> 3 *co-codamol tablets 8/500*

3.80 Which of the following would be inappropriate for a GP to prescribe on an NHS prescription?

> 1 *Altacite Plus® tablets*
> 2 *Halycitrol® emulsion*
> 3 *Senokot® tablets*

3.81 Which of the following would a pharmacist be reimbursed for if dispensed against an NHS prescription?

1 Accu-Chek Active® meter
2 Ferraris Pocketpeak® peak flow meter
3 Melgisorb® sterile dressings size 10 cm × 10 cm

3.82 Which of the following is allowed on an NHS dental prescription?

1 cefradine capsules
2 erythromycin capsules
3 flucloxacillin capsules

3.83 A report should be made to the Committee on Safety of Medicines for which of the following adverse reactions?

1 anaphylaxis caused by a drug marketed for 15 years
2 development of a rash following treatment with a new antibiotic
3 severe CNS effects following administration of a vaccine

3.84 Which of the patients presenting prescriptions for the following items would normally be exempt from paying NHS prescription charges?

1 a 22-year-old woman with a prescription for Cerazette®
2 a 50-year-old woman with a prescription for Elleste-Solo® 1 mg tablets
3 a 54-year-old woman with a prescription for Progynova® tablets

3.85 Which of the following classes of patients are exempt from paying NHS prescription charges?

1 a 33-year-old quadriplegic man with a prescription for flucloxacillin capsules
2 a 42-year-old woman with insulin-dependent diabetes mellitus with a prescription for ramipril tablets
3 a 47-year-old employed man with a prescription for carbimazole tablets

3.86 NHS prescriptions for clobazam capsules are permissible if they are endorsed with 'SLS' and used to treat:

1 acute alcohol withdrawal
2 anxiety (short-term use)
3 epilepsy

3.87 Which of the following proprietary medicines should display cautionary label 8 when dispensed?

1 Asmabec Clickhaler®
2 Inderal-LA®
3 Zyloric®

3.88 Which of the following conditions would an NHS contractor have to fulfil for entitlement to payment for additional professional services?

1 display up to a maximum of eight health promotion leaflets
2 keep patient medication records
3 produce a practice leaflet

Section IV   *6 questions*

The following questions consist of two statements. Choose as your answer, from A to E, which of the following is appropriate. (*For Answers, see Chapter 7.*)

> A: *both statements are true and the second statement is a correct explanation of the first statement*
> B: *both statements are true, but the second statement is not a correct explanation of the first statement*
> C: *the first statement is true but the second statement is false*
> D: *the first statement is false but the second statement is true*
> E: *both statements are false*

3.89 **1st statement:** a type C vaginal contraceptive cap (Vimule Cap®) and Delfen® may be obtained from a medical practitioner on an NHS prescription

2nd statement: contraceptive products listed in the Drug Tariff are allowed on NHS prescriptions

3.90 **1st statement:** Viaflex® or Steriflex® containers must be used to administer glyceryl trinitrate infusions

2nd statement: glyceryl trinitrate is incompatible with polyvinyl chloride containers

3.91 **1st statement:** omeprazole tablets should carry the cautionary label: 'Do not take indigestion remedies at the same time as this medicine'

2nd statement: enteric coatings may be damaged by antacids

3.92 **1st statement:** it is good practice, when providing domiciliary oxygen services, to have adequate communication channels with the patient's GP and/or respiratory unit

2nd statement: pharmacists should monitor the progress of treatment of patients and inform the doctor of any problems when supplying domiciliary oxygen

3.93 **1st statement:** certain foods may be prescribed on an NHS prescription for patients with cystic fibrosis

2nd statement: the Advisory Committee on Borderline Substances approves certain foods for specific clinical conditions

Question 3.94 concerns the following prescription:

> *10 chloroquine 250 mg tabs*
> *500 mg stat, then 500 mg b.d.*

3.94 **1st statement:** this medicine may be sold rather than have the prescription dispensed

2nd statement: chloroquine 250 mg tablets, when used as malaria prophylaxis, are Pharmacy (P) medicines

Pharmacy Law and Ethics

All candidates undertaking the preregistration examination require an understanding of pharmacy law. However, much of the daily running of a pharmacy is not directly defined by statute law, but rather from the development of good practice and fulfilling the guidance stated in 'Medicines, Ethics and Practice: a Guide for Pharmacists'.

Legislation relating to pharmacy can be difficult to comprehend. A suitable approach would be to read the whole of Medicines, Ethics and Practice: a Guide for Pharmacists and think about how the law applies during your working practice of pharmacy, as well as asking pharmacists about their interpretation (of pharmacy law).

Tables 4.1 and 4.2, and Figure 4.1, summarise information that preregistration candidates would be expected to know, and may be examined in the actual exam. Practice questions follow the summaries.

Poisons schedules

A non-medicinal poison is defined as a substance included on the poisons list of the Poisons Act 1972, which comprises two parts:

- Part I poisons: substances on this list are sold by persons lawfully conducting retail pharmacy businesses, i.e. sales of Part I

Table 4.1 Pharmacy law and ethics topics which preregistration candidates are expected to understand

- Aspects of prescribing
- Dispensing
- Controlled drugs regulations
- POMs/P medicines/GSL medicines
- Poisons Act 1972
- Methylated Spirits Regulations 1987
- Responsibilities of a pharmacist (ethics)
- Standards of professional practice

Table 4.2 Legal requirements of controlled drugs

Requirement	Schedule 2 (CD)	Schedule 3 (CD No Reg)	Schedule 4, Part I (CD Benz)	Schedule 4, Part II (CD Anab)	Schedule 5 (CD Inv)
Examples	Diamorphine, morphine, methadone	Benzphetamine, buprenorphine, temazepam	Nitrazepam, loprazolam, flurazepam	Nandrolone	Low-strength codeine
Safe custody	Yes (except secobarbital)	All exempt, except buprenorphine, diethylpropion, flunitrazepam, temazepam	No	No	No
Prescription requirements	Yes	Yes, except temazepam	No	No	No
Handwriting requirements	Yes	Yes, except phenobarbital and temazepam	No	No	No
Requisitions necessary	Yes	Yes	No	No	No
Entry into CD register	Yes	No	No	No	No
Emergency supplies allowed	No	No, except phenobarbital	Yes	Yes	Yes
Repeats allowed on prescriptions	No	No	Yes	Yes	Yes
Invoices retained for 2 years	No	Yes	No	No	Yes
UK address for prescriber	Yes	Yes	No	No	No
Licences required for import and export	Yes	Yes	Yes	Yes (unless in the form of a medicine and for self-administration)	No
Validity of prescription	13 weeks	13 weeks	6 months	6 months	6 months

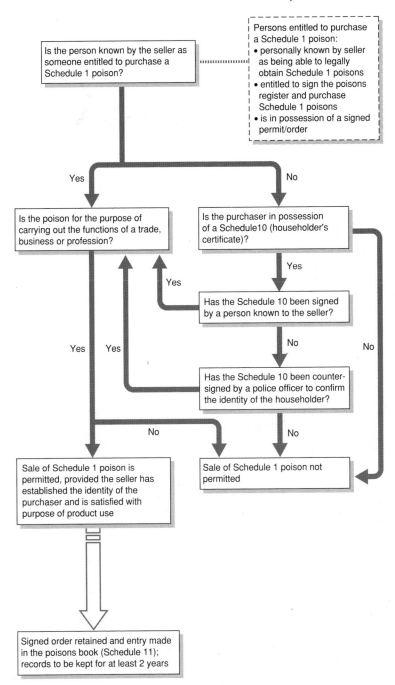

Figure 4.1 Procedures involved in the sale of Schedule 1 poisons.

poisons must be made through registered pharmacies under the supervision of a pharmacist.

● Part II poisons: substances on this list may be sold by persons able to sell Part I poisons and by listed sellers of Part II poisons (maintained by a local authority).

Poisons are categorised into Schedules as specified by the Poisons Rules 1982, as amended. The Poisons Amendment Order 1985 removed Schedules 2, 3, 6 and 7. The eight Schedules are briefly described below:

Schedule 1   A list of poisons where special restrictions are applied to the storage, conditions sale and the need to retain the records of sale

Schedule 4   A list of substances which are exempt from control as poisons

Schedule 5   A list of Part II poisons which may be sold by listed sellers

Schedule 8   Application form for inclusion in the local authority's sellers list of Part II poisons

Schedule 9   Form retained by a local authority of the list of listed sellers of Part II poisons

Schedule 10   Certificate enabling the purchase of a non-medicinal poison

Schedule 11   Entry form made in the poisons book regarding the sale of Schedule 1 poison

Schedule 12   Form of authority required for the purchase of certain poisons, e.g. strychnine

Professional judgement

Pharmacists are expected to exercise a greater duty of care compared to most other professionals, due to their extensive knowledge and training. The working day of a practising pharmacist involves constant decision-making, which is often not easy.

Professional judgement is based on experience, knowledge and assessment of the consequences of feasible options. Figure 4.2 provides a summary of the factors involved in choosing a particular course of action.

Section I

STYLE 1 – SIMPLE COMPLETION TYPE

Select the most appropriate answer for each of the following questions or incomplete statements. (*For Answers, see Chapter 7.*)

4.1 Which one of the following non-prescription medicines has the least abuse potential?

A: *cyclizine tablets*
B: *loratadine tablets*
C: *kaolin and morphine mixture*
D: *surgical spirit*
E: *senna tablets*

4.2 Mrs F regularly takes citalopram tablets 20 mg daily and requests an emergency supply of such medication, as she has currently run out. What is the maximum number of citalopram 20 mg tablets that may be lawfully supplied?

A: 0
B: 5
C: 7
D: 14
E: 28

4.3 A man comes into your pharmacy requesting the emergency hormonal contraceptive (morning-after-pill) for his girlfriend. He states that unprotected intercourse occurred 4 days ago. The girlfriend is not present at the pharmacy. You should refuse the request because:

A: *no attempt has been made to contact a doctor*
B: *levonorgestrel is not licensed for use after 72 hours (3 days) of unprotected intercourse*
C: *you have not personally interviewed the patient*
D: *you do not know the patient*
E: *you do not know the man*

4.4 Which one of the following is acceptable practice when dispensing unlicensed medicines?

A: *allowed in hospital pharmacies only*
B: *allowed only in pharmacies with special licences*
C: *allowed if prescribed by a doctor for a named patient*
D: *allowed only for products of specified legal categories*
E: *never allowed*

4.5 Which of the following is the final available option for preventing or controlling exposure to a hazardous substance, based on the COSHH Regulations 1998?

A: *elimination of the use of the substance*
B: *handle the substance in an isolation cabinet*
C: *substitution with a less hazardous form of the substance*
D: *substitution with a different and less hazardous substance*
E: *wearing suitable protective clothing*

4.6 Which one of the following is not a requirement for the emergency supply of a Prescription Only Medicine?

A: *the label must state 'emergency supply'*
B: *the pharmacist must interview the patient*
C: *the patient should state their name and address*
D: *the patient should state the name and address of the pharmacy that made the last supply of their required medicine*
E: *a record of the emergency supply must be made*

4.7 Which one of the following is essential for computerised patient medication records?

A: *inform the local pharmaceutical committee*
B: *inform the local general practitioners*
C: *inform patients by advertising through local newspapers*
D: *inform the primary care trust*
E: *register with the Data Protection Commission*

4.8 Which one of the following applies to medicines taken by patients into hospital?

A: *become the property of the hospital*
B: *must be destroyed by the nursing staff*
C: *must be destroyed by the patient or their relatives*
D: *must be destroyed by a hospital pharmacist*
E: *remains the property of the patient*

4.9 The prime concern of the pharmacist is:

A: *adhering to relevant law and regulations*
B: *co-operating with other health professionals*
C: *providing an efficient pharmaceutical service*
D: *staying up-to-date with pharmaceutical knowledge*
E: *the welfare of the patient and public*

4.10 Which one of the following is not a concern of the Royal Pharmaceutical Society of Great Britain?

A: *definition of standard of conduct for pharmacists*
B: *implement disciplinary procedures for misdemeanours associated with the sale of medicines and poisons by pharmacists*
C: *maintenance of the register of pharmaceutical chemists*
D: *provision of a benevolent fund for pharmacists*
E: *represent pharmacists in trade disputes*

4.11 How many members are there in the Council of the Royal Pharmaceutical Society of Great Britain?

A: *10*
B: *15*
C: *20*
D: *21*
E: *24*

Section II

STYLE 2 – CLASSIFICATION TYPE

For each question select the appropriate lettered option. The letter options within a group of questions may be used once, more than once, or not used. (*For Answers, see Chapter 7.*)

Questions 4.12 to 4.18 concern the following:

    A: *British National Formulary*
    B: *Drug Tariff*
    C: *Labelling on the packaging of commercially produced medicines*
    D: *Martindale*
    E: *Medicines, Ethics and Practice: a Guide for Pharmacists*

Which one of the above would be an appropriate source of information for the following situations?

4.12 Determining the legal status of a medicinal product   E

4.13 Storage of controlled drugs as required by UK legislation   E

4.14 Contact telephone numbers for drug information services   ·

4.15 Whether a medicinal product may be sold within the UK

4.16 A report form for suspected adverse drug reactions   )

4.17 Determining payment for maintaining patient records

4.18 Ascertaining the number of NHS prescription charges for a particular medicinal product

Section III

STYLE 3 – MULTIPLE COMPLETION TYPE

Three responses accompany each question. Choose as your answer, from A to E, which of the following is appropriate. (*For Answers, see Chapter 7.*)

> A: *1, 2 and 3 are correct*
> B: *1 and 2 correct only*
> C: *2 and 3 correct only*
> D: *1 correct only*
> E: *3 correct only*

4.19 Which of the following non-repeatable prescriptions, dated 5 months previously, are not legally valid?

1 *a prescription for atenolol tablets*
2 *a prescription for co-codamol tablets*
3 *a prescription for fentanyl patches*

4.20 Which of the following are applicable to a patient requesting an emergency supply of a medicine?

1 *any medicines may be requested by the patient for an emergency supply*
2 *items dispensed for an emergency supply are free of charge*
3 *the requesting patient must be personally interviewed by the pharmacist*

4.21 Which of the following is not in keeping with the philosophy of continuing professional development (CPD) for pharmacists?

1 *attending as many professional courses as possible to fulfil the CPD quota*
2 *designing activities that meet individual learning and development needs*
3 *reflecting on personal practice in order to identify areas that may be improved*

4.22 Which of the following applies to a pharmacy premises?

1 *compliance with the Health and Safety at Work Act with regard to employees and customers*
2 *COSHH regulations with respect to medicinal products*
3 *a written policy on health and safety if there are more than five employees*

4.23 Prescriptions for temazepam tablets may:

1 *be computer-generated but signed in ink by the prescriber*
2 *have the direction 'as directed'*
3 *use a date stamp by the prescriber*

4.24 Audits:

1 *are always conducted internally by the service provider*
2 *are a means for improving the standard of service*
3 *focus on an aspect of service*

4.25 Which of the following must be complied with when obtaining pethidine injections from a wholesaler?

1 *an entry must be made in the controlled drugs register when receiving the supply*
2 *pethidine injections must be stored in a controlled drugs cabinet*
3 *the quantity of pethidine injections must be stated in words and figures on a written order to the wholesaler*

4.26 Which of the following controlled drugs would require a prescription to be written in the prescriber's own handwriting?

1 *Oramorph® oral solution 10 mg/5 ml (Schedule 5 controlled drug)*
2 *methylphenidate tablets 10 mg (Schedule 2 controlled drug)*
3 *oxycodone tablets 5 mg (Schedule 2 controlled drug)*

4.27 Which of the following are true about clinical governance?

1 *audits and continuing professional development may be involved*
2 *identifies the person(s) accountable for the overall quality of care*
3 *controlling expenditure is part of clinical excellence*

4.28 Electronic patient medication records:

1 *are allowed to be inspected immediately by the patient if they so desire*

2 *do not have to be registered under the Data Protection Act 1998*

3 *may have a fee levied to the patient requesting the information kept*

4.29 Diamorphine tablets may be prescribed in which of the following situations?

1 *by a licensed medical practitioner for the treatment of drug addiction*

2 *by a general practitioner for the symptomatic relief of pain*

3 *by a registered nurse practitioner for the symptomatic relief of pain*

4.30 Which of the following should be recorded in an accident book?

1 *the gender of the injured person*

2 *the occupation of the injured person*

3 *any measures taken to prevent recurrence*

4.31 Which of the following conditions apply to diazepam tablets?

1 *require storage in the controlled drugs cabinet*

2 *prescription must state in words and figures the amount to be supplied*

3 *prescription must include the age of the patient, if under 12 years old*

4.32 The Health and Safety at Work Act 1974 compels a pharmacy manager to:

1 *ensure that all machinery is maintained*

2 *provide appropriate training information and training for employees to safely carry out their duties*

3 *ensure safe storage and transportation of articles and substances*

4.33 Which of the following applies to medicines, except controlled drugs, handed to a pharmacy by a patient?

1 *returned to stock if it is still in date and has no evidence of tampering*

2 *its destruction must be witnessed by an agent acting on behalf of the police or Royal Pharmaceutical Society of Great Britain*

3 *dispatched to the assigned authority for the destruction of special waste*

4.34 Which of the following conditions apply to phenobarbital tablets?

1 *the prescription must state the age of the patient, if under 12 years old*

2 *the prescription must state the quantity to be dispensed in words and figures*

3 *the prescription must state the dose of phenobarbital to be taken*

4.35 The code of ethics is:

1 *an all-inclusive guide detailing all aspects of a pharmacist's professional conduct and practice*

2 *a requirement of the Medicines Act 1968*

3 *applicable to the behaviour of pharmacists, whether they practice pharmacy or not*

The following questions consist of two statements. Choose as your answer, from A to E, which of the following is appropriate. (*For Answers, see Chapter 7.*)

> A: both statements are true and the second statement is a
>   correct explanation of the first statement
> B: both statements are true, but the second statement is not a
>   correct explanation of the first statement
> C: the first statement is true but the second statement is false
> D: the first statement is false but the second statement is true
> E: both statements are false

4.36 **1st statement:** the use of patient medication record data, in an anonymous form, for research would constitute professional misconduct

2nd statement: in most instances, information presented in a confidential manner must be respected and protected

4.37 **1st statement:** prescriptions may be lawfully handed out while the pharmacist is away on lunch-break

2nd statement: a retail pharmacy remains under the personal control of a pharmacist, and personal control does not cease if the pharmacist is absent for a very short period of time

4.38 **1st statement:** standard operating procedures are used by staff to accurately carry out particular tasks

2nd statement: a pharmacist must always write the standard operating procedures

4.39 **1st statement:** the Data Protection Commissioner should be informed if personal data are to be kept by the pharmacy in the form of patient medication records

2nd statement: it is a criminal offence to process personal data without notifying the Data Protection Commissioner

4.40 **1st statement:** medicinal products should be obtained from a reputable source

2nd statement: a pharmacist should ensure that the medicines they supply are of an acceptable quality

4.41 Mrs J takes phenobarbital tablets 60 mg each night for partial seizures and has three tablets remaining. She has given her repeat prescription to her GP surgery but comes into your pharmacy asking for an emergency supply of phenobarbital, in case her doctor does not issue a new prescription in time.

1st statement: an emergency supply should not be made in this case

2nd statement: phenobarbital is classified as a Schedule 3 controlled drug

Open book questions

STYLE 1 – SIMPLE COMPLETION TYPE

Select the most appropriate answer for each of the following questions or incomplete statements. (*For Answers, see Chapter 7.*)

4.42 Which of the following OTC medicines may have a self-selection or prominent open display within the pharmacy?

A: *32 aspirin 300 mg tablets*
B: *24 aspirin 400 mg and codeine 8 mg tablets*
C: *16 paracetamol 500 mg tablets*
D: *12 paracetamol 500 mg, caffeine 30 mg and codeine 8 mg tablets*
E: *24 ibuprofen 200 mg tablets*

4.43 An emergency supply may be made of which of the following?

A: *DHC Continus® tablets 60 mg*
B: *Oramorph® concentrated oral solution 100 mg/5 ml*
C: *OxyNorm® capsules 5 mg*
D: *Pallidone SR® capsules 5 mg*
E: *Temgesic® tablets 200 micrograms*

4.44 Which one of the following does not have to be stored in the controlled drugs cabinet?

A: *buprenorphine tablets 200 micrograms*
B: *Diconal® tablets*
C: *methylphenidate tablets 10 mg*
D: *morphine mixture 1 mg/ml*
E: *morphine sulphate oral solution 10 mg/5 ml*

4.45 It is a requirement for a pharmacist to endorse which one of the following on an NHS prescription, when dispensing a Schedule 2 or 3 controlled drug?

A: *CD*
B: *date of supply*
C: *manufacturer of dispensed product*
D: *quantity supplied*
E: *pack size*

4.46 What is the maximum amount of industrial methylated spirit a medical practitioner may obtain on one signed order?

A: *1 litre*
B: *2 litres*
C: *3 litres*
D: *10 litres*
E: *20 litres*

Section II

For each question select the appropriate lettered option. The letter options within a group of questions may be used once, more than once, or not used. (*For Answers, see Chapter 7.*)

Questions 4.47 and 4.48 relate to the following controlled drugs:

A: *diazepam tablets 2 mg*
B: *phenobarbital tablets 30 mg*
C: *morphine sulphate oral solution 10 mg/5 ml*
D: *morphine sulphate concentrated oral solution 100 mg/5 ml*
E: *temazepam tablets 20 mg*

Select, from A to E, which one of the above:

4.47 Does not need a licence for export and import

4.48 Requires the patient's name and address to be written in the prescriber's own handwriting

Questions 4.49 to 4.51 concern the following drugs:

A: *amobarbital*
B: *buprenorphine*
C: *fentanyl*
D: *methadone*
E: *phenobarbital*

Which one of the above applies to the following statements?

4.49 May be dispensed as an 'emergency supply'

4.50 Is exempt from the safe custody requirements but not the handwriting requirements

4.51 Is exempt from the handwriting requirements but not the safe custody requirements

Questions 4.52 and 4.53 concern the following:

A: 0.02%
B: 0.2%
C: 1.0%
D: 1.5%
E: 2.0%

To be classified as a CD Inv P, the following preparations must not exceed which one of the above strengths?

4.52 Morphine in a liquid preparation

4.53 Single-dose preparations of pholcodine which are not for parenteral use

Three responses accompany each question. Choose as your answer, from A to E, which of the following is appropriate. (*For Answers, see Chapter 7.*)

> A: *1, 2 and 3 are correct*
> B: *1 and 2 correct only*
> C: *2 and 3 correct only*
> D: *1 correct only*
> E: *3 correct only*

4.54 Guidance regarding standard operating procedures (SOPs) for dispensing include:

> 1 *the pharmacist responsible for the daily operation of the pharmacy should normally direct the development of SOPs*
> 2 *it is recommended that SOPs be reviewed at least every 2 years*
> 3 *SOPs are not required where no support staff exist*

4.55 Which of the following statements apply to veterinary medicines?

> 1 *the type of animal to be treated must be stated on the dispensing label*
> 2 *the prescription must have a declaration stating that the medicine is for an animal or herd under the care of the veterinary surgeon*
> 3 *the pharmacist must supervise the sale of pharmacy and merchant veterinary medicines when conducted in a pharmacy*

4.56 Regarding the provision of services to drug addicts, which of the following are correct?

> 1 *sugar-free methadone liquid may be supplied on a prescription specifying the syrup formulation*
> 2 *patient medication records must be used and notified to the Information Commissioner*
> 3 *pharmaceutical services may be declined to drug addicts if their behaviour is considered unacceptable*

4.57 The holder of a certificate of proficiency of ambulance paramedic skills may administer which of the following parenteral prescription-only medicines?

1 atropine sulphate
2 dihydrocodeine tartrate
3 sodium chloride

4.58 In which of the following situations may confidential information about patients be disclosed without their consent?

1 the request of the parent(s) of an adolescent
2 the request of a coroner
3 to prevent serious injury to the patient or to others associated with the patient

4.59 Guidance on prescription delivery services states that:

1 the pharmacist must deliver the medicines
2 delivery arrangements should be made between the pharmacist and the patient or carer
3 records should be kept for each delivery

4.60 Which of the following are correct with respect to paracetamol?

1 the retail sale of paracetamol tablets must be labelled with 'if symptoms persist, consult your doctor'
2 amounts greater than 32 tablets of paracetamol 500 mg can be supplied only with a valid prescription
3 children under the age of 12 cannot use paracetamol

4.61 Opticians in the course of their professional practice, or emergency, may be sold or supplied which of the following products?

1 chloramphenicol eye ointment 1%
2 hypromellose eye drops 0.3%
3 tropicamide eye drops 0.5%

4.62 Pharmacists should make the Royal Pharmaceutical Society of Great Britain aware of which of the following?

1 if the professional competence of another pharmacist is placing the public at risk
2 if there are any circumstances that prevent them from offering any particular service
3 if they are unable to work for a period of 12 weeks or longer

4.63 Which of the following products should not be sold from a pharmacy?

1 *alcoholic beverage*
2 *tobacco products for non-medicinal use*
3 *lottery tickets*

4.64 The Chemical (Hazard Information and Packaging) 2 Regulations 1995 (CHIP 2) specify:

1 *chemicals are classified before supply*
2 *hazardous chemicals are labelled with appropriate risk and safety phrases*
3 *a safety data sheet should be provided with all sales for public domestic use*

4.65 The labelling of containers and packaging of manufactured medicinal products for human use must include:

1 *date of manufacture*
2 *expiry date*
3 *pharmaceutical form of the product*

Section IV

STYLE 4 – ASSERTION–REASON TYPE

The following questions consist of two statements. Choose as your answer, from A to E, which of the following is appropriate. (*For Answers, see Chapter 7.*)

A: *both statements are true and the second statement is a correct explanation of the first statement*
B: *both statements are true, but the second statement is not a correct explanation of the first statement*
C: *the first statement is true but the second statement is false*
D: *the first statement is false but the second statement is true*
E: *both statements are false*

4.66 **1st statement:** emergency supplies of buprenorphine are allowed in certain circumstances

2nd statement: buprenorphine is a Schedule 3 controlled drug

4.67 **1st statement:** strychnine must be supplied in its original packaging

2nd statement: strychnine is a Schedule 1 poison

4.68 **1st statement:** pethidine injections are allowed to be supplied by one midwife to another midwife

2nd statement: midwives may possess and administer pethidine injections in the course of their duties

5

Responding to Symptoms

A major role of the community pharmacist is to be able to assess and recommend solutions to common healthcare problems that the general public may encounter. Furthermore, diagnosis and management of minor ailments is a significant proportion of the preregistration examination.

The best method of preparation for responding to symptoms is to practise using actual situations within the community environment, and at the earliest opportunity. Each consultation should help candidates to develop a good questioning technique, an appreciation of the appropriateness of OTC products, and confidence about the advice given to patients.

Tables 5.1–5.10 and Figures 5.1–5.6 summarise information that-preregistration candidates would be expected to know, and may be examined in the actual exam. Practice questions follow the summaries.

Table 5.1 Responding to symptoms: topics likely to occur in the preregistration examination

Candidates are expected to know how to recognise and treat the following minor ailments:
• Pain (acute pain, musculoskeletal, period pains)
• Headaches and migraines
• Topical infections (athlete's foot, threadworms, headlice)
• Coughs and colds (flu, sore throats, coughs)
• Gastrointestinal problems (nausea and vomiting, diarrhoea, constipation, dyspepsia)
• Genitourinary conditions (cystitis, thrush)
• Allergies (hayfever, skin allergies)
• Skin conditions (acne, cold sores, warts, corns, calluses)
• Children's illness (meningitis, colic, nappy rash)
• Emergency hormonal contraception
• Smoking cessation
• First aid

Table 5.2 Types of OTC products that require additional considerations regarding their use

1. Recent POM to P changes, e.g. omeprazole, simvastatin
2. Medicines with interaction problems, e.g. antacids
3. Medicines and substances liable to misuse, e.g. citric acid, kaolin and morphine mixture, Phenergan® elixir
4. Excessive quantities of any medicine, e.g. paracetamol, senna
5. Products that have a common ingredient, e.g. paracetamol, antihistamines

Table 5.3 Aspirin and NSAIDs

Things to remember:

- aspirin and NSAIDs can cause GI problems (avoid in stomach ulcers) and worsening asthma
- aspirin should not be given to children and adolescents under 16 years due to risk of Reye's syndrome
- pregnant women and asthmatics should consult their doctor before taking aspirin or ibuprofen
- patients' allergic to aspirin may also be sensitive to ibuprofen
- care required in recommending products with paracetamol – risk of paracetamol overdose
- aspirin and NSAIDs commonly interact with warfarin, lithium and methotrexate

Table 5.4 Ingestion remedies

Things to remember

- determine whether patient is suffering from indigestion and not constipation or diarrhoea
- magnesium-containing antacids have a laxative effect
- aluminium-containing antacids can lead to constipation
- preparations with a high content of sodium can worsen hypertension or cardiac failure
- side-effects of H_2 antagonists include GI disturbances, headache, rash and dizziness
- refer to GP if symptoms persist after 2 weeks

Table 5.5 Topical hydrocortisone (up to 1% w/w)

Things to remember

- may be sold on its own without prescription for the following indications: mild to moderate eczema; allergic contact dermatitis; irritant dermatitis; and insect bite reactions
- may be sold in combined preparations for the following: athlete's foot and candidial intertrigo (hydrocortisone + clotrimazole or miconazole); and in anal and perianal itching associated with haemorrhoids (hydrocortisone + lignocaine)
- OTC contraindications: not for use on eyes, face (except ears), ano-genital region, broken or infected skin, children under 10 years, and pregnant women
- applied sparingly over a small area once or twice daily for up to 7 days

Table 5.6 Allergy symptoms that require referral to a medical practitioner

Symptoms	Possible diagnosis
Erythema around the mouth and nose with weeping vesicles and yellow-brown crusted scabs	Infective eczema or impetigo
Butterfly-shaped reddening over nose and cheeks	Acne rosacea or SLE
Rash on one side of the face, scalp or skin around the eye	Shingles
Red and oedematous rash on previously healthy skin	Cellulitis
Symptoms not responding to OTC treatments	Severe symptoms

Table 5.7 Thrush and vaginitis

Refer to doctor if the patient presents with any of the following:
- first-time sufferers
- more than two attacks in the previous 6 months
- pregnant and breast-feeding mothers
- girls under 16 years and women over 60
- blood-stained vaginal discharge or irregular vaginal bleeding
- abdominal pain
- problems with micturition
- fever
- gastrointestinal disturbance (diarrhoea, nausea, vomiting)
- ulcers or blisters on the vagina or vulva
- previous history of STD
- no improvement after 7 days

Table 5.8 Vitamins

Vitamin	Function in the body	Dietary sources
A (retinal)	Regeneration of membranes Formation of light-sensitive substances in the eye	Dairy products, egg yolks, liver, oily fish, broccoli, carrots, tomatoes
B_1 (thiamine)	Breakdown of carbohydrates, nerve cell function	Yeast, liver, cereals, milk, eggs
B_2 (riboflavine)	Oxidation processes, including respiration	Yeast, liver, cereals, milk, eggs
B_6 (pyridoxine)	Protein metabolism	Eggs, wholemeal flour, fish
B_{12} (cyanocobalamin)	Blood production	Liver, liver extracts, meat, fish, eggs

Continued

Table 5.8 Vitamins—Cont'd

Vitamin	Function in the body	Dietary sources
Nicotinic acid (part of the B complex)	Enzyme systems	Meat, fish, wholemeal flour
C (ascorbic acid)	Modulating the body's immune system; formation, maintenance and repair of intercellular cement material; absorption of iron in vegetarians	Citrus fruit, berries, green vegetables
D (calciferol)	Calcium metabolism and bone formation	Fish liver oil, animal fats, dairy produce
E (tocopherol)	Antioxidant properties, may be important for normal neurological function	Nuts, vegetables
K (phytomenadione)	Blood clotting factors	Green vegetables, liver

Table 5.9 Minerals

Mineral	Function in the body	Dietary sources
Iron	Required for the formation of haemoglobin	Red meat, liver, green vegetables, cereals
Calcium	Formation and maintenance of bones and teeth	Milk, cheese, yoghurt, vegetables, nuts
Phosphorus	Aids calcium to make bones strong and rigid; essential for healthy nerves	Meat, milk, dairy products, nuts
Magnesium	Required for functioning of heart and nervous system; aids calcium for production of healthy bones	Bread, wholegrain cereals, green vegetables
Sodium	Essential for nerve and muscle function and fluid balance	Salt, processed foods
Potassium	Required for functioning of muscles and nerves, and maintaining fluid balance and blood pressure	Fruit, vegetables, bread, cereals, meat
Zinc	Required for immune system, healthy sperm, growth, taste, smell and insulin release; component of enzymes	Meat, shellfish, milk, dairy produce
Copper	Essential for healthy food and nerves	Meat, fish, cereals, green vegetables, pulses
Selenium	Component of antioxidant enzyme; essential for healthy prostate gland and sperm	Brazil nuts, cereals, meat, liver

Table 5.10 Normal and abnormal body temperatures (measured orally)

Normal	37°C ± 0.5°C
Fever	> 38.5°C
Child high fever	> 40°C
Adult high fever	> 41°C

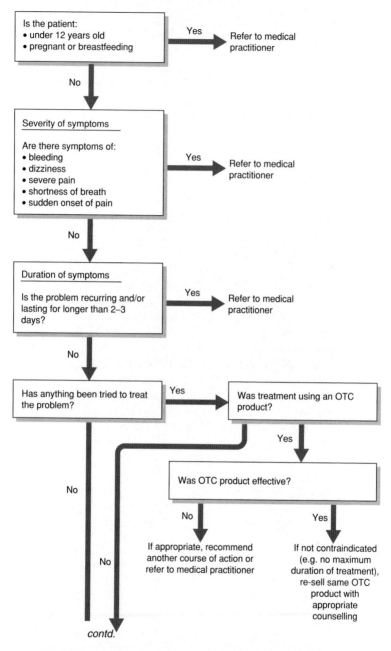

Figure 5.1 Responding to symptoms: summary of the general principles.

Continued

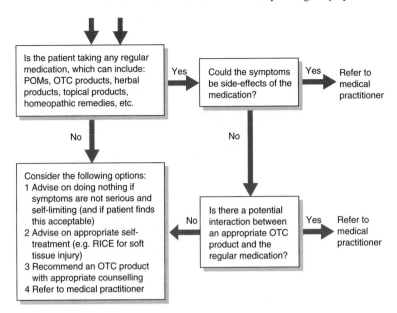

Figure 5.1 Cont'd

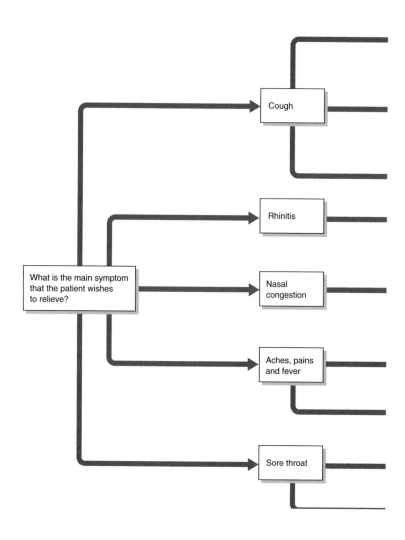

Figure 5.2 Summary of OTC product recommendations for coughs and colds.

Continued

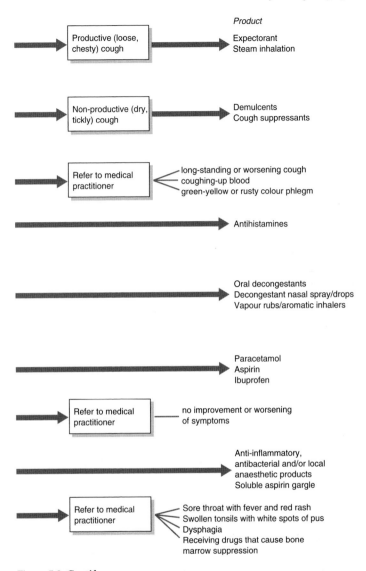

Product

Productive (loose, chesty) cough → Expectorant
Steam inhalation

Non-productive (dry, tickly) cough → Demulcents
Cough suppressants

Refer to medical practitioner ← long-standing or worsening cough
coughing-up blood
green-yellow or rusty colour phlegm

→ Antihistamines

→ Oral decongestants
Decongestant nasal spray/drops
Vapour rubs/aromatic inhalers

→ Paracetamol
Aspirin
Ibuprofen

Refer to medical practitioner — no improvement or worsening of symptoms

→ Anti-inflammatory, antibacterial and/or local anaesthetic products
Soluble aspirin gargle

Refer to medical practitioner ← Sore throat with fever and red rash
Swollen tonsils with white spots of pus
Dysphagia
Receiving drugs that cause bone marrow suppression

Figure 5.2 Cont'd

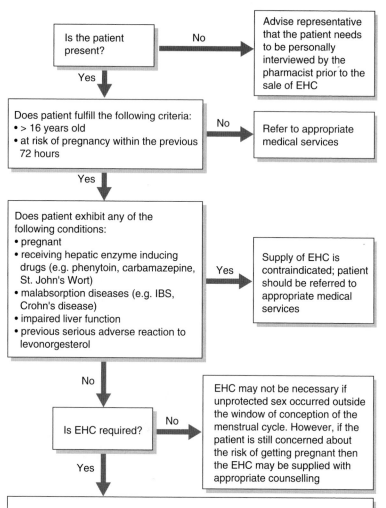

Figure 5.3 Summary of the pharmacist procedure for supplying the emergency hormonal contraceptive (EHC).

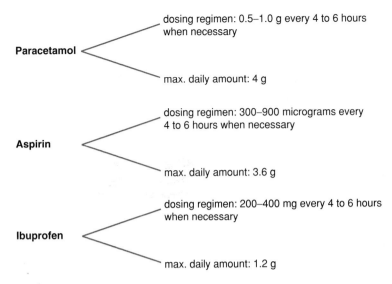

Figure 5.4 Simple adult analgesic doses.

Paracetamol
- dosing regimen: 0.5–1.0 g every 4 to 6 hours when necessary
- max. daily amount: 4 g

Aspirin
- dosing regimen: 300–900 micrograms every 4 to 6 hours when necessary
- max. daily amount: 3.6 g

Ibuprofen
- dosing regimen: 200–400 mg every 4 to 6 hours when necessary
- max. daily amount: 1.2 g

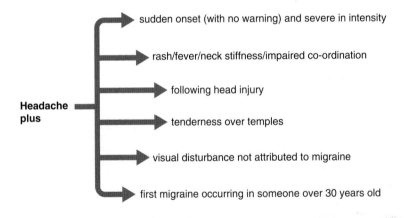

Headache plus
- sudden onset (with no warning) and severe in intensity
- rash/fever/neck stiffness/impaired co-ordination
- following head injury
- tenderness over temples
- visual disturbance not attributed to migraine
- first migraine occurring in someone over 30 years old

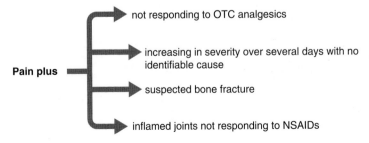

Pain plus
- not responding to OTC analgesics
- increasing in severity over several days with no identifiable cause
- suspected bone fracture
- inflamed joints not responding to NSAIDs

Figure 5.5 Headache and pain symptoms that require referral to a medical practitioner.

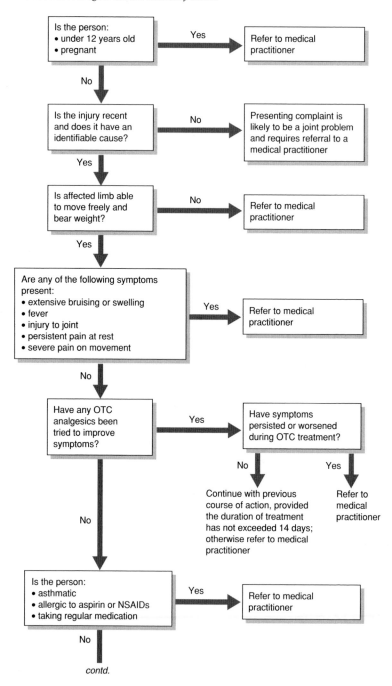

Figure 5.6 Protocol for muscular aches, sprains and backache.

Continued

OTC product options:
- Oral NSAIDs may be recommended to reduce inflammation and pain;
- Topical NSAIDs or rubefacients are suitable alternatives to oral NSAIDs, provided the area affected does not have broken skin
- Paracetamol may be equally effective as NSAIDs in reducing musculoskeletal pain (e.g. low back pain)

Counselling
1 General advice is to rest musculoskeletal injuries
2 For acute low back pain, it is recommended that there should be minimal or no bed rest with a return to normal activities as soon as possible
3 Referral to medical practitioner is required if symptoms worsen or do not improve within 5 days of starting treatment

Figure 5.6 Cont'd

Section I

STYLE 1 – SIMPLE COMPLETION TYPE

Select the most appropriate answer for each of the following questions or incomplete statements. (*For Answers, see Chapter 7.*)

5.1 To which one of the following would it be appropriate to sell hydrocortisone cream 1%?

A: *an 8-month-old child with nappy rash*
B: *an 8-year-old child with insect bites*
C: *a woman with a rash on her face*
D: *a woman with a rash on her wrist caused by an allergy to metal*
E: *a man with dermatitis self-treating with hydrocortisone cream 1% for the previous 5 weeks*

5.2 A 34-year-old woman comes into your pharmacy complaining of widespread itching over her body which started 10 days ago, after returning from Algeria. She has a yellow-brown tanned complexion, and also states that she feels 'run down' and has trouble sleeping. She has not tried any self-treatment. Which of the following is an appropriate recommendation for her current condition?

A: *use an antihistamine*
B: *use calamine lotion*
C: *use hydrocortisone cream 1%*
D: *use a soap substitute (e.g. emulsifying ointment)*
E: *refer to her GP*

5.3 Chloroquine and proguanil may be purchased without prescription for use as malarial prophylaxis. What is the recommended duration of treatment?

A: *1 week before entering an endemic area and at least 4 weeks after leaving*

B: *1 week before entering an endemic area and at least 6 weeks after leaving*

C: *2 weeks before entering an endemic area and at least 4 weeks after leaving*

D: *2 weeks before entering an endemic area and at least 6 weeks after leaving*

E: *4 weeks before entering an endemic area and at least 4 weeks after leaving*

5.4 The following are symptoms of a specific childhood illness:

- *rash which is red-brown in colour and widespread, covering the neck, face and upper chest*
- *high temperature*
- *nasal discharge and conjunctivitis*
- *complains of aching limbs*
- *white spots surrounded by a red ring present in the mouth*

These symptoms are suggestive of:

A: *allergy to certain foods*

B: *chicken-pox*

C: *measles*

D: *mumps*

E: *rubella*

5.5 Beclometasone nasal spray is available as a Pharmacy (P) medicine to adults over the age of 18 years. For which one of the following conditions could an appropriate sale be made?

A: *allergic rhinitis*

B: *common cold symptoms*

C: *epistaxis*

D: *nasal polyps*

E: *sinusitis*

5.6 Skin lesions circular in shape with well-defined edges and central healing are characteristic of which one of the following infections:

A: *atopic eczema*
B: *contact eczema*
C: *impetigo*
D: *psoriasis*
E: *ringworm*

5.7 Risk factors for developing coronary heart disease do not include:

A: *diabetes*
B: *high intake of fat*
C: *hypertension*
D: *irritable bowel syndrome*
E: *lack of physical activity*

5.8 The recommended minimum age in an infant for changing from formula milk to cow's milk is:

A: *4 months*
B: *6 months*
C: *12 months*
D: *18 months*
E: *24 months*

5.9 Women planning to become pregnant should ensure that they have immunity to rubella. This is because:

A: *pregnancy predisposes to rubella infections*
B: *rubella can cause fetal malformations during the early stages of pregnancy*
C: *rubella increases the risk of miscarriage during pregnancy*
D: *rubella develops into a more serious condition during pregnancy*
E: *rubella may cause infertility in women of child-bearing age*

5.10 Which one of the following would be appropriate for treating fungal infections involving the toenail?

A: *OTC clotrimazole cream 1% applied to the affected area*
B: *OTC fluconazole capsule 150 mg taken for 1 day*
C: *OTC potassium permanganate solution used to soak the affected foot*
D: *OTC zinc undecenoate powder applied to both feet*
E: *referred to GP for a prescription-only medicine*

5.11 Which one of the following would not necessitate a recommendation for a GP referral?

A: *an asthmatic increasing the use of a salbutamol inhaler*
B: *an infant with wheeze*
C: *a man recovering from a cold but complaining of a dry, tickly cough*
D: *a man with a persistent cough who has regular enalapril tablets*
E: *a woman with a persistent cough who smokes 30 cigarettes a day*

5.12 Mr Q presents to your pharmacy with a bright red patch in the white of his right eye. There is no pain or visual disturbance, and the pupils respond to light and are of equal size. He has no recent history of trauma or head injury. You should recommend which one of the following?

A: *use an antibacterial eye preparation (e.g. propamidine eye drops)*
B: *use an astringent eye preparation (e.g. zinc sulphate eye drops)*
C: *refer to an optometrist for an eye test*
D: *refer to a GP for a prescription-only medicine*
E: *no treatment is required*

5.13 To which one of the following is it appropriate to sell OTC cimetidine tablets 100 mg?

A: *a child of 10 years of age*
B: *a 23-year-old smoker*
C: *a 28-year-old pregnant woman*
D: *a 30-year-old man on phenytoin*
E: *a 30-year-old man on warfarin*

5.14 Which of the following fish contains a high content of omega-3 marine triglycerides?

A: *cod*
B: *halibut*
C: *haddock*
D: *mackerel*
E: *plaice*

5.15 Which of the following are likely to present with oral candidiasis?

A: *a 10-year-old boy who takes salbutamol syrup*
B: *a 17-year-old woman with mouth ulcers*
C: *a 30-year-old woman who breast-feeds her infant*
D: *a 40-year-old man who smokes*
E: *a 60-year-old man who wears ill-fitting dentures*

5.16 Asthmatics complaining of cold symptoms, and presenting with increasing coughing and wheezing, should be recommended the following:

A: *an explanation that antibiotics are the best treatment for a common cold*
B: *an explanation that no treatment is necessary*
C: *referral to a medical practitioner*
D: *use of a decongestant that does not contain phenylpropanolamine*
E: *use of paracetamol to treat cold symptoms*

5.17 Which one of the following is not an expectorant?

A: *ammonium chloride*
B: *chlorphenamine*
C: *citric acid*
D: *guaiphenesin*
E: *ipecacuanha*

5.18 Bacterial conjunctivitis has which one of the following signs or symptoms?

A: *itchiness*
B: *dislike of light*
C: *pain*
D: *sticky yellow discharge*
E: *swelling*

5.19 Which one of the following can be appropriately recommended for an OTC purchase?

   A: *aspirin for a headache experienced by a 10-year-old child*
   B: *codeine linctus for a chesty, productive cough*
   C: *hydrocortisone cream for acne*
   D: *ibuprofen for an aspirin-sensitive individual*
   E: *miconazole gel for an infant with oral thrush*

5.20 Miconazole cream 2% may be used to treat fungal skin infections. Treatment should be continued for how many additional days after the lesions have healed?

   A: *1 day*
   B: *3 days*
   C: *5 days*
   D: *7 days*
   E: *10 days*

5.21 Which one of the following could be used with paracetamol as additional analgesia?

   A: *co-codamol*
   B: *co-codaprin*
   C: *co-dydramol*
   D: *co-proxamol*
   E: *Migraleve®*

Section II

STYLE 2 – CLASSIFICATION TYPE

For each question select the appropriate lettered option. The letter options within a group of questions may be used once, more than once, or not used. (*For Answers, see Chapter 7.*)

Questions 5.22 to 5.24 concern the following:

> A: *hyoscine butylbromide tablets 10 mg*
> B: *ibuprofen tablets 200 mg*
> C: *paracetamol tablets 500 mg*
> D: *pseudoephedrine tablets 60 mg*
> E: *senna tablets 7.5 mg*

> Select, from A to E, which one of the above is not suitable for people with the following conditions.

5.22 Asthma

5.23 Pyloric stenosis

5.24 Hypertension

Questions 5.25 to 5.27 concern the following conditions:

> A: *cold sores*
> B: *impetigo*
> C: *scabies*
> D: *shingles*
> E: *urticaria*

> Select, from A to E, which one of the above relates to the following statements.

5.25 All members of the household should be treated if one person presents with signs or symptoms of this condition

5.26 It begins as small red lumps that develop into minute blisters, resulting in a characteristic rash over the face, scalp or trunk

5.27 It is a contagious bacterial infection

Questions 5.28 to 5.33 concern the following vitamins:

> A: *folic acid*
> B: *vitamin B*$_{12}$
> C: *vitamin C*
> D: *vitamin D*
> E: *vitamin E*

Select, from A to E, which vitamin applies to the following statements.

5.28 Autoimmune gastritis results in malabsorption of this vitamin

5.29 Exists in vegetable oils

5.30 Increases intestinal absorption of calcium

5.31 Increases absorption of iron from plant sources

5.32 Synthesised in skin during exposure to sunlight

5.33 Its intake is recommended prior to, and during, the first 12 weeks of pregnancy

Questions 5.34 to 5.37 concern the following actions:

> A: *advise the patient to undertake appropriate lifestyle modifications*
> B: *advise that no treatment is necessary as the condition is self-limiting*
> C: *advise on the use of an OTC preparation and to go to the GP if the symptoms have not improved in 7 days*
> D: *advise on the use of an OTC preparation and to go to the GP if the symptoms have not improved in 3 days*
> E: *advise to make an appointment with the GP*

Select, from A to E, which one of the above is the appropriate action for the following.

5.34 A 47-year-old man has suffered with a hoarse voice for the past 6 weeks. He has been using antiseptic lozenges but these have not improved his condition

5.35 A 62-year-old man would like a product to treat his haemorrhoids, which has previously been diagnosed and treated by his GP

5.36 A 23-year-old woman complains of the frequent urge to pass urine, which is painful. She also states that she has a fever and pain in the groin

5.37 A 30-year-old man has aching back pain after doing some gardening work. He describes the pain as irritating and has not taken any medication for it

Questions 5.38 to 5.40 concern the following products:

> A: *azelastine hydrochloride 140 micrograms/dose nasal spray*
> B: *pseudoephedrine tablets 60 mg*
> C: *sodium chloride 2% nasal spray*
> D: *terfenadine tablets 60 mg*
> E: *xylometazone 0.1% nasal spray*

Select, from A to E, which of the above applies to the following statements.

5.38 Reduces the effects of beta-blockers

5.39 May cause cardiac arrhythmias if taken at excessive dosage

5.40 Optimum therapeutic effect occurs after 2–3 weeks of continuous treatment

Questions 5.41 and 5.42 relate to the following options for diarrhoea:

> A: *ispaghula husk*
> B: *kaolin and morphine mixture*
> C: *loperamide capsules 2 mg*
> D: *oral rehydration therapy*
> E: *refer to a GP*

Which one of the above would be an appropriate option?

5.41 Acute diarrhoea in a 1-year-old child in the previous 6 hours

5.42 Acute diarrhoea in a 30-year-old woman who has recently returned from South America

Questions 5.43 to 5.45 concern the following minerals:

    A: *calcium*
    B: *iron*
    C: *potassium*
    D: *selenium*
    E: *zinc*

Which one of the above:

5.43 Is involved in the metabolism of carbohydrates and is the main cation of intracellular fluid   c

5.44 May be deficient if there is a lack of vitamin D   A

5.45 Is absorbed more readily from plant sources through the action of vitamin C

STYLE 3 – MULTIPLE COMPLETION TYPE

Three responses accompany each question. Choose as your answer, from A to E, which of the following is appropriate. (*For Answers, see Chapter 7.*)

> A: *1, 2 and 3 are correct*
> B: *1 and 2 correct only*
> C: *2 and 3 correct only*
> D: *1 correct only*
> E: *3 correct only*

5.46 Dreemon® (diphenhydramine hydrochloride 25 mg) tablets are used for temporary relief of sleeplessness. An appropriate sale may be made to which of the following people?

1 *an 18-year-old man having trouble sleeping and is due to travel by plane in 3 days*
2 *a 32-year-old man in good general health who has had his sleep disrupted due to a change in his work pattern*
3 *a 62-year-old woman with type 2 diabetes mellitus who has sleep disturbance following a flight from Canada*

5.47 Meningitis exhibits which of the following symptoms?

1 *headache*
2 *neck stiffness*
3 *vomiting*

5.48 Women at high risk of having a child with a neural tube defect include:

1 *a woman receiving anti-epileptic drugs*
2 *a woman who has a child with a neural tube defect*
3 *a woman whose partner has spina bifida*

5.49 The side-effects of hyoscine include:

1 *dry mouth*
2 *diarrhoea*
3 *insomnia*

5.50 To which of the following would it be inappropriate to sell Canesten Thrush Cream® (clotrimazole 2%) without the need of a prescription?

1 *a woman who is pregnant*
2 *a woman who is 14 years old*
3 *a woman who is experiencing her first episode of vaginal candidiasis*

5.51 Which of the following would require a referral to the GP?

1 *a schoolboy presenting with athlete's foot*
2 *a man presenting with cystitis*
3 *a man with type 2 diabetes mellitus presenting with bunions and corns on the feet*

5.52 Which of the following statements applies to the treatment of threadworms?

1 *affected persons should wash their hands and scrub their nails prior to eating*
2 *mebendazole is suitable for those over 2 years of age*
3 *every member of the household should be treated*

5.53 Constipation may be caused by:

1 *hyoscine butylbromide*
2 *morphine sulphate*
3 *magnesium trisilicate*

5.54 Which of the following drugs would require additional contraceptive precautions if the woman also receives a regular oral contraceptive?

1 *carbamazepine*
2 *phenytoin*
3 *omeprazole*

5.55 Which of the following may be used for treating any aspect of migraine?

1 *metoclopramide*
2 *paracetamol with buclizine and codeine*
3 *pizotifen*

5.56 Referral to a GP would be appropriate for which of the following cold symptoms?

  1 nasal congestion
  2 chest pain during breathing
  3 shortness of breath

5.57 The whole household should be treated in:

  1 chickenpox
  2 ringworm
  3 threadworms

5.58 Referral to a GP would be appropriate for which of the following symptoms?

  1 vomit that is dark brown in colour
  2 feeling nauseous
  3 loss of appetite over the previous day

5.59 For which of the following conditions is smoking a risk factor?

  1 bronchitis
  2 coronary heart disease
  3 peptic ulcer

5.60 Which of the following applies to classical migraine?

  1 occurs more in men than women
  2 some relief may be obtained by lying in a darkened room
  3 sufferers may experience altered vision at the start of an attack

5.61 Hydrocortisone cream 1% may be sold without a prescription for:

  1 contact dermatitis on the leg
  2 insect bites on the leg
  3 irritant dermatitis on the face

5.62 Women who are pregnant should avoid:

  1 contact with cat litter
  2 eating liver
  3 eating soft unpasteurised cheese

5.63 Children under 16 years of age, except on the advice of a doctor, should not use which of the following?

1 aspirin
2 ibuprofen
3 paracetamol

5.64 Which of the following are inappropriate first aid procedures for a recently acquired blister burn on the palm of a hand?

1 apply a sterile, non-adhesive dressing
2 apply an antiseptic ointment
3 use a sterile needle to burst the blister

5.65 Which of the following questions should be asked if a person wishes to purchase treatment for head lice?

1 is any member of the household asthmatic
2 how many and what are the ages of the children of the household
3 have head lice been observed on any member of the household

Section IV

STYLE 4 – ASSERTION–REASON TYPE

The following questions consist of two statements. Choose as your answer, from A to E, which of the following is appropriate. (*For Answers, see Chapter 7.*)

> A: *both statements are true and the second statement is a correct explanation of the first statement*
> B: *both statements are true, but the second statement is not a correct explanation of the first statement*
> C: *the first statement is true but the second statement is false*
> D: *the first statement is false but the second statement is true*
> E: *both statements are false*

5.66 **1st statement:** pharmacists should advise customers of contraception methods when making a sale of emergency hormonal contraception

2nd statement: emergency hormonal contraception is licensed to be used only once within one menstrual cycle

5.67 **1st statement:** parasiticidal shampoo is more effective than a parasiticidal lotion for the treatment of head lice

2nd statement: alcohol-based head lice products are not recommended for use by asthmatics

5.68 **1st statement:** three portions of fruit and vegetables is the recommendation for reducing the risk of developing cancer

2nd statement: fruit and vegetables contain antioxidants which help to counteract the build-up of free radicals within the body

5.69 **1st statement:** pregnant women are recommended to take cod-liver supplements

2nd statement: the risk of miscarriage is reduced by increasing the intake of vitamin A

5.70 **1st statement:** a folic acid supplement should be taken during the first trimester of pregnancy

2nd statement: folic acid levels may be reduced in pregnant women who smoke

5.71 **1st statement:** nicotine chewing gum should be chewed for up to 5 minutes

2nd statement: the maximal amount of nicotine is released within the first 5 minutes of chewing

5.72 **1st statement:** pregnant women should eat large amounts of liver and vitamin-A-containing foods during the first trimester

2nd statement: liver is rich in vitamin A

5.73 **1st statement:** the treatment for the removal of verrucae may involve salicyclic-acid-containing products

2nd statement: verrucae are caused by a viral infection

5.74 **1st statement:** vegans may use yeast extract as a supplement to their diet

2nd statement: vegans may not derive sufficient amounts of vitamin B_{12} from their diet

5.75 **1st statement:** oral rehydration salts are not an appropriate treatment for diarrhoea in people with type 1 diabetes mellitus

2nd statement: intestinal absorption of sodium and water is increased by the glucose content of oral rehydration salts

Style 1 – Simple completion type

Select the most appropriate answer for each of the following questions or incomplete statements. (*For Answers, see Chapter 7.*)

5.76 Zantac 75® is licensed for the self-treatment of indigestion symptoms for up to:

A: *3 days*
B: *5 days*
C: *7 days*
D: *10 days*
E: *14 days*

5.77 Pavacol D® should not be sold to which of the following patients?

A: *a woman who breast-feeds her infant*
B: *a woman who takes Colpermin® capsules*
C: *a woman who takes Yasmin® tablets*
D: *a woman who takes metformin tablets*
E: *a woman who takes Ventolin Evohaler® and Becotide®-100 inhaler*

5.78 To which one of the following would it be appropriate to allow the sale of Piriton Allergy® tablets?

A: *a man taking amiodarone*
B: *a man with epilepsy*
C: *a woman with glaucoma*
D: *a man with prostate problems*
E: *a woman with severe liver disease*

5.79 Which one of the following would be appropriate for prophylaxis against malaria in Honduras for a family of two adults and two children (aged 9 and 11)?

A: *advice from the GP should be sought for the whole family*
B: *malarial prophylaxis is not required*
C: *chloroquine should be taken by the whole family*
D: *chloroquine should be taken by the adults, but advice from the GP should be sought for the children*
E: *chloroquine and proguanil should be taken by the whole family*

5.80 How should a person use Sudafed Decongestant Nasal Spray®?

A: *twice a day for a maximum of 5 days*
B: *four times a day for a maximum of 5 days*
C: *two or three times a day for a maximum of 7 days*
D: *four times a day for a maximum of 7 days*
E: *twice a day for a maximum of 10 days*

5.81 Which of the following would be appropriate for treating head-lice in children with asthma?

A: *Carylderm® liquid*
B: *Derbac-M® liquid*
C: *Full Marks® lotion*
D: *Prioderm® lotion*
E: *Lyclear Dermal® cream*

5.82 Mr N comes into your pharmacy and asks you to recommend something for an 'upset stomach'. He takes antihypertensive medication. Which one of the following could you recommend?

A: *Algicon® suspension*
B: *Altacite Plus® suspension*
C: *Gaviscon® liquid*
D: *Macrogel®*
E: *magnesium trisilicate mixture BP*

5.83 Treatment of gingivitis is not an indication for which one of the following?

A: *Corsodyl® dental gel*
B: *Corsodyl® mouthwash*
C: *Difflam® oral rinse*
D: *Eludril® mouthwash*
E: *Oraldene®*

5.84 Which one of the following products should be avoided by a person with dyspepsia?

A: *Paracodol®*
B: *Propain®*
C: *Solpadeine®*
D: *Syndol®*
E: *Veganin®*

5.85 What is the first option for treating acute diarrhoea?

A: *antibiotics*
B: *antispasmodics*
C: *kaolin and morphine mixture*
D: *loperamide*
E: *oral rehydration preparations*

Section II

For each question select the appropriate lettered option. The letter options within a group of questions may be used once, more than once, or not used. (*For Answers, see Chapter 7.*)

Questions 5.86 and 5.87 concern the following OTC products:

   A: *Joy-Rides*®
   B: *Phenergan*®
   C: *Sea-Legs*®
   D: *Stugeron 15*®
   E: *Valoid*®

   Select, from A to E, which one of the above:

5.86 Is the most sedating anti-emetic for travel sickness

5.87 Has the quickest onset of action for the prevention of motion sickness

Questions 5.88 to 5.90 concern the following:

   A: *cyproheptadine*
   B: *buclizine*
   C: *clemastine*
   D: *chlorphenamine*
   E: *promethazine*

   Which of the above:

5.88 Is an ingredient in an OTC preparation for the relief of migraine

5.89 Is an OTC product with an indication for correction of temporary sleep disturbance

5.90 Has an indication for migraine

Questions 5.91 to 5.93 concern the following preparations:

A: *Aludrox® liquid*
B: *Asilone® suspension*
C: *Gavison® liquid*
D: *sodium bicarbonate powder*
E: *Milk of Magnesia®*

Select, from A to E, which preparation is appropriate for the following conditions:

5.91 Relief of abdominal discomfort resulting from trapped wind

5.92 Relieves indigestion and constipation

5.93 Protects against heartburn and reflux oesophagitis

Questions 5.94 to 5.96 concern the following topical preparations:

A: *Conotrane cream*
B: *hydrocortisone butyrate 0.1% cream*
C: *hydrocortisone 1% cream*
D: *tacalcitol ointment*
E: *terbinafine cream*

Select which of the above preparations:

5.94 Is applied to the affected area in fungal skin infections

5.95 May be purchased without prescription for treating nappy rash

5.96 Is indicated for the treatment of severe forms of eczema

Section III

Style 3 – Multiple completion type

Three responses accompany each question. Choose as your answer, from A to E, which of the following is appropriate. (*For Answers, see Chapter 7.*)

>   A: *1, 2 and 3 are correct*
>   B: *1 and 2 correct only*
>   C: *2 and 3 correct only*
>   D: *1 correct only*
>   E: *3 correct only*

5.97 Which of the following may be taken by a patient on ACE inhibitors?
> 1 *Candiden*® *vaginal tablet*
> 2 *potassium citrate mixture*
> 3 *Sudafed Dual Relief Non-Drowsy*® *capsules*

5.98 Which of the following medicines would require women to take more than 400 micrograms of folic acid before and during pregnancy?
> 1 *carbamazepine*
> 2 *fluoxetine*
> 3 *sulpiride*

5.99 Which of the following should be avoided in a patient with hyperthyroidism?
> 1 *aspirin*
> 2 *Piriton Allergy*® *tablets*
> 3 *Do-Do Chesteze*® *tablets*

5.100 Which of the following analgesics may be used by a woman in her first trimester?
> 1 *aspirin*
> 2 *ibuprofen*
> 3 *paracetamol*

5.101 A person with epilepsy may take which of the following?

1 *piperazine*
2 *paracetamol*
3 *pseudoephedrine*

5.102 Which of the following should be avoided by a patient taking Betopic® ophthalmic solution?

1 *Kwells® tablets*
2 *Piriton Allergy® tablets*
3 *Rynacrom® 4% nasal spray*

5.103 Oral sympathomimetic decongestants are not recommended in which of the following conditions?

1 *diabetes mellitus*
2 *hypertension*
3 *glaucoma*

Section IV   *4 questions*

The following questions consist of two statements. Choose as your answer, from A to E, which of the following is appropriate. (*For Answers, see Chapter 7.*)

> A: both statements are true and the second statement is a correct explanation of the first statement
> B: both statements are true, but the second statement is not a correct explanation of the first statement
> C: the first statement is true but the second statement is false
> D: the first statement is false but the second statement is true
> E: both statements are false

5.104 **1st statement:** Pavacol D® is suitable for a dry tickly cough in a person with diabetes mellitus

2nd statement: Pavacol D® is a preparation that is sugar-free and has an antitussive action

Questions 5.105 and 5.106 concern the following situation. Mr B hands in a prescription for amitriptyline tablets 50 mg and wants to buy some Piriton Allergy® tablets for hay fever.

5.105 **1st statement:** a pharmacodynamic interaction can exist between amitriptyline and chlorphenamine

2nd statement: antimuscarinic side-effects are exhibited by amitriptyline and chlorphenamine

5.106 **1st statement:** Benadryl Allergy Relief® tablets are a suitable alternative to Piriton Allergy® tablets for Mr B

2nd statement: antimuscarinic side-effects are less common with non-sedating antihistamines

5.107 **1st statement:** Canestan Oasis® would be inappropriate for a woman taking methenamine tablets

2nd statement: methenamine requires the urine to be acidic in its activity

6 *Calculations*

One of the essential requirements for passing the preregistration examination is to obtain at least 70% (or 14 out of 20 questions) in the calculations section of the open book paper. Pharmacists should have the ability to carry out calculations, without the need for a calculator, for the following reasons:

- performing accurate calculations is an essential skill in the practice of pharmacy;
- the use of calculators increases the risk of arithmetical errors, which can lead to fatal incidents;
- and the absence of calculators helps to develop a 'sense of number' to recognise errors.

Preparation for the calculation section begins by forbidding the use of calculators throughout the period of preregistration training. The general approach to calculation is as follows:

1. Determine what information is known and what needs to be obtained from reference sources (for the purpose of the exam this is the BNF);
2. Convert units if required;
3. Simplifying the calculation by manipulating the appropriate mathematical formula to scale-up, scale-down or substitute numbers;
4. Simplifying the calculation by cancelling of numbers.

The key to a successful pass mark is to practise calculation questions, as much and as often as possible.

Tables 6.1–6.6 and Figure 6.1 summarise information that preregistration candidates would be expected to know, and may be examined in the actual exam. Practice questions follow the summaries.

Table 6.1 Arithmetical techniques examined during the preregistration examination

- Fractions
- Percentages
- Decimals
- Parts
- Cancelling
- Addition/Subtraction/Multiplication/Division
- Scaling up and down of doses/formulae/concentrations

Table 6.2 Concentrations of chloroform water

	% v/v of chloroform	Dilution required to make single-strength chloroform water
Chloroform water (single strength)	0.25	–
Double-strength chloroform water	0.5	1:1
Concentrated chloroform water	10	1:40
Chloroform spirit	5	1:20

Table 6.3 Concentrations of peppermint water

	% v/v of peppermint oil	Dilution required to make single-strength peppermint water
Peppermint water (single strength)	0.05	–
Concentrated peppermint water	2	1:40
Concentrated peppermint emulsion	2	1:40
Peppermint spirit	10	1:200

Table 6.4 Units of mass

Unit	Expression	Amount equivalent to 1 kg
kilogram	kg	1 kg
gram	g	1000 g
milligrams	mg	1×10^6 mg
micrograms	mcg or μg	1×10^9 micrograms
nanograms	ng	1×10^{12} ng

Table 6.5 Units of volume

Unit	Expression	Amount equivalent to 1 litre
litre	l	1 litre
millilitre	ml	1000 ml
microlitre	μl	1×10^6 μl

Table 6.6 Concentration terms

Unit	Expression	Example
% weight in weight	% w/w	1% w/w = 1 g in 100 g
% weight in volume	% w/v	1 % w/v = 1 g in 100 ml
% volume in volume	% v/v	1 % v/v = 1 ml in 100 ml
1 part in 10 parts	1 in 10	10 parts in total
1 part to 10 parts	1:10	11 parts in total
1 part per 100 (solid in solid)	1 in 100	1 in 100 = 1 g in 100 g = 1 % w/w
1 part per 100 (solid in liquid)	1 in 100	1 in 100 = 1 g in 100 ml = 1 % w/v
1 part per 100 (liquid in liquid)	1 in 100	1 in 100 = 1 ml in 100 ml = 1 % v/v
molar	M	1 molar = 1 mole in 1 litre

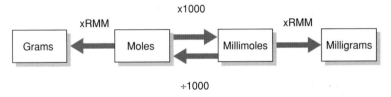

Figure 6.1 Converting expressions of mass.

$$1 \text{ mol} = x \text{ g}$$
$$1 \text{ mmol} = x \text{ mg}$$

Questions

Some questions will require the use of the BNF, others will not.

Section I   15 questions

Select the most appropriate answer for each of the following
questions or incomplete statements. (*For Answers, see Chapter 7.*)

6.1 How much concentrated rose water is required to prepare 400
ml of equal parts rose water to witch hazel?

A: 2.5 ml
B: 4 ml
C: 5 ml
D: 40 ml
E: 100 ml

6.2 How much sodium chloride should be added to 400 g of water
to produce a 10% w/w solution?

A: 44.4 mg
B: 444 mg
C: 44.4 g
D: 360 g
E: 444 g

6.3 What weight of menthol would be required to prepare 600 g of
0.25% w/w menthol in aqueous cream?

A: 0.5 mg
B: 1.5 mg
C: 5 g
D: 15 g
E: 150 g

6.4 A dermatologist requests an extemporaneous preparation of 100 g of hydrocortisone 0.8% cream. How much 2.5% hydrocortisone cream is required for this preparation?

A: *3.2 g*
B: *4 g*
C: *25 g*
D: *32 g*
E: *40 g*

6.5 How much of 0.5% w/v stock solution is required to produce 2 litres of a 1 in 8000 solution?

A: *2.8 ml*
B: *16 ml*
C: *50 ml*
D: *64 ml*
E: *80 ml*

6.6 Fersamal® syrup is given to a premature infant at a dose of 2.4 ml/kg daily. The infant weighs 2.0 kg. What is the daily dose of ferrous iron received by the infant?

A: *4.8 mg*
B: *43.2 mg*
C: *48 mg*
D: *134.4 mg*
E: *224 mg*

6.7 What single dose of Fucidin® suspension should be given to a 3-month-old infant weighing 5.4 kg?

A: *1.8 ml*
B: *2.2 ml*
C: *2.7 ml*
D: *4.0 ml*
E: *5.4 ml*

6.8 Mrs L is on the intensive care unit and is given the following fluids in a 24-hour period:

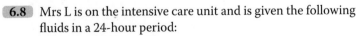

- 1 litre of glucose 5% infusion over 8 hours
- 1 litre of NaCl 0.9% infusion containing 20 mmol KCl over 8 hours
- 1 litre of KCl, NaCl and glucose intravenous infusion containing 20 mmol KCl over 8 hours

How much glucose has Mrs L received in 24 hours?

A: 9 g
B: 27 g
C: 90 g
D: 180 g
E: 270 g

6.9 10 ml of water is required to dissolve 1 g of sodium bicarbonate. What is the strength, in w/w, of the resulting saturated solution? (1 ml of water is equivalent to 1 g.)

A: 4.54%
B: 9.09%
C: 10%
D: 10.9%
E: 11.1%

6.10 500 g of an ointment containing 12.5% w/w of emulsifying wax is prepared. The weight of emulsifying wax in 280 g of ointment is:

A: 9.6 g
B: 22.0 g
C: 26.8 g
D: 29.0 g
E: 35.0 g

6.11 The specification for a tablet containing a labelled content of 200 mg of active ingredient states that the tablet contains between 90 and 110% of that active ingredient. The limits of the tablet's content is:

A: 100–200 mg
B: 160–180 mg
C: 180–220 mg
D: 195–205 mg
E: 200–240 mg

6.12 A 14-year-old is staying in Armenia for 2 weeks in July. Chloroquine cannot be supplied due to a manufacturing problem. How many proguanil 100 mg tablets should be dispensed for prophylaxis against malaria?

A: 28

B: 49

C: 70

D: 98

E: 112

6.13 What volume of Bricanyl® syrup is equivalent to the active ingredient in one Bricanyl® tablet?

A: 5 ml

B: 10 ml

C: 12.5 ml

D: 15 ml

E: 16.67 ml

6.14 How much potassium permanganate would be needed to prepare 1 litre of a 1 in 200 solution?

A: 200 mg

B: 500 mg

C: 1 g

D: 2.5 g

E: 5 g

6.15 You receive the following prescription:

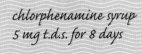

chlorphenamine syrup
5 mg t.d.s. for 8 days

What quantity of chlorphenamine oral solution should you supply?

A: 70 ml
B: 100 ml
C: 200 ml
D: 250 ml
E: 300 ml

Section II

STYLE 2 – CLASSIFICATION TYPE

For each question select the appropriate lettered option. The letter options within a group of questions may be used once, more than once, or not used. (*For Answers, see Chapter 7.*)

Questions 6.16 and 6.17 concern the following quantities:

A: *0.04 mg*
B: *0.4 mg*
C: *4 mg*
D: *40 mg*
E: *400 mg*

Select, from A to E, which one of the above:

6.16 Is the weight of loratadine in 40 ml loratadine syrup

6.17 Is the weight of KCl in 100 ml of a 0.4% solution

Questions 6.18 and 6.19 concern the following quantities of potassium citrate powder:

A: *0.02 g*
B: *0.2 g*
C: *2 g*
D: *20 g*
E: *200 g*

Select, from A to E, the amount required for the following preparations:

6.18 200 ml of a 1 in 1000 solution of potassium citrate

6.19 4 litres of a 0.05% solution of potassium citrate

Questions 6.20 to 6.22 concern the following doses:

A: *50 mg q.d.s.*
B: *60 mg t.d.s.*
C: *100 mg t.d.s.*
D: *100 mg q.d.s.*
E: *150 mg q.d.s.*

Which one of the above doses applies to the following situations?

6.20 The upper limit of an ibuprofen single dose for treating juvenile arthritis in a 1-year-old child

6.21 The recommended minimum intramuscular dose of clindamycin for a 4-year-old child with a severe infection

6.22 The usual intramuscular dose of cefuroxime for a new born baby weighing 3 kg

Questions 6.23 and 6.24 concern the following quantities of sodium bicarbonate:

A: 0.3 g
B: 3 g
C: 30 g
D: 300 g
E: 3000 g

Select, from A to E, the amount used for preparing:

6.23 600 ml of aromatic magnesium carbonate mixture BP

6.24 60 ml of kaolin and morphine mixture BP

Questions 6.25 and 6.26 concern the following quantities of sodium:

A: 1 mmol
B: 10 mmol
C: 100 mmol
D: 150 mmol
E: 1000 mmol

Select, from A to E, which of the above applies to the following statements.

6.25 The sodium content must be less than what value for tablets to be termed 'low Na^+'

6.26 How many mmol is equivalent to 60 g of sodium chloride present in physiological saline

Section III

Three responses accompany each question. Choose as your answer, from A to E, which of the following is appropriate. (*For Answers, see Chapter 7.*)

> A: *1, 2 and 3 are correct*
> B: *1 and 2 correct only*
> C: *2 and 3 correct only*
> D: *1 correct only*
> E: *3 correct only*

6.27 Which of the following is equivalent to 0.3 mg?

1 *0.03 ml of a 1 in 10 000 solution*
2 *0.3 ml of a 1 in 1000 solution*
3 *3 ml of a 100 microgram/ml solution*

6.28 Which of the following doses, given every 4 hours, are within BNF recommended limits for a 5-year-old child receiving pentazocaine by subcutaneous injection?

1 *0.5 ml of the 30 mg/ml injection*
2 *0.7 ml of the 30 mg/ml injection*
3 *1.0 ml of the 30 mg/ml injection*

6.29 Which of the following doses, for the relief of acute pain, are within BNF recommended limits for a 3-year-old child receiving pethidine by intramuscular injection?

1 *0.8 ml of a 10 mg/ml injection*
2 *0.3 ml of a 50 mg/ml injection*
3 *0.6 ml of a 50 mg/ml injection*

6.30 Which of the following is equivalent to calcium 500 mg daily?

1 *Calcichew® tablets 1 o.d.*
2 *Calcium-Sandoz® syrup 5 ml t.d.s.*
3 *Ossopan® tablets 1 o.d.*

6.31 Which of the following is equivalent to ferrous iron 200 mg daily?

1 *2 Fersaday® tablets*
2 *2 Feospan® capsules*
3 *2 Fersamal® tablets*

Section IV

The following questions consist of two statements. Choose as your answer, from A to E, which of the following is appropriate. (*For Answers, see Chapter 7.*)

> A: both statements are true and the second statement is a correct explanation of the first statement
> B: both statements are true, but the second statement is not a correct explanation of the first statement
> C: the first statement is true but the second statement is false
> D: the first statement is false but the second statement is true
> E: both statements are false

6.32 **1st statement:** the infusion rate for a 0.2% lidocaine infusion may be set at 120 ml/hour for the initial 30 minutes

2nd statement: the recommended rate of infusion of lidocaine is 4 mg/minute for the first 30 minutes following the bolus dose

6.33 **1st statement:** 3 litres of 8.4% w/v sodium bicarbonate give 3000 mmol each of sodium and bicarbonate ions

2nd statement: sodium bicarbonate 8.4% w/v contains 1 mmol/ml of electrolytes

6.34 An injection contains 25 mg of active ingredient in a 12.5 ml ampoule
1st statement: the strength of the solution is 20% w/v

2nd statement: 1 ml contains 2 mg of active ingredient

7 Answers

2 Clinical pharmacy and therapeutics: closed book

Section I   *23 answers*

Style 1 – Simple completion type

2.1 Answer D

The administration of tetracyclines and iron salts at the same time may result in both drugs having decreased gut absorption and lower drug serum levels. [Refer to BNF Appendix 1 (interactions).]

2.2 Answer D

The international normalised ratio (INR) is used to establish the maintenance dose of warfarin. The INR target for atrial fibrillation is 2.5. The main adverse effect of all oral anticoagulants is haemorrhage. The British Society for Haematology recommends a reduction or withdrawal of warfarin dose when the INR is less than 6.0 units but more than 0.5 units above target value. [Refer to BNF 2.8.2 (oral anticoagulants).]

2.3 Answer E

BMI = weight (kg)/height (m)^2.

BMI ranges:
<20 = underweight
20–25 = desired range
25–30 = overweight
>30 = obese

2.4 Answer B

Side-effects include throbbing headache, flushing, dizziness and postural hypotension, as a result of vasodilatation of blood vessels by nitrates. [Refer to BNF 2.6.1 (nitrates).]

2.5 **Answer C**

A 5-HT$_1$ agonist is appropriate for treating an acute migraine attack when simple analgesics are ineffective. The other drugs mentioned are for prophylaxis, chronic recurrent attacks or only for hospital use. [Refer to BNF 4.7.4.1 (treatment of the acute migraine attack).]

2.6 **Answer D**

The action of statins is to competitively inhibit HMG CoA reductase, a liver enzyme involved in cholesterol synthesis. Statins are recommended to be taken at night because maximal cholesterol synthesis occurs at night. Atorvastatin may be taken at any time of the day. [Refer to BNF 2.12 (lipid-regulating drugs).]

2.7 **Answer D**

Phenothiazines are dopamine antagonists and prevent nausea and/or vomiting by blocking the chemoreceptor trigger zone. The other classes of drug can cause nausea and/or vomiting. [Refer to BNF 4.6 (drugs used in nausea and vertigo).]

2.8 **Answer A**

Beta-blockers should be avoided as they can precipitate asthma – antagonism of beta$_2$-receptors causes constriction of the bronchial airways.

2.9 **Answer C**

Maintenance therapy with antipsychotic depot injections is a recognised alternative if compliance with oral medication is a problem. Injections are given at intervals of 1 to 4 weeks. The dose and dosage interval are titrated according to the response of the patient. [Refer to BNF 4.2.2 (administration of antipsychotic depot injections).]

2.10 **Answer C**

Ketoprofen is a non-steroidal anti-inflammatory drug (NSAID). Bleeding is a serious upper gastrointestinal side-effect associated with all NSAIDs. [Refer to BNF 10.1.1 (non-steroidal anti-inflammatory drugs).]

2.11 Answer D
Corticosteroids are interchangeable for emergency treatment, and the equivalent anti-inflammatory dose of suitable corticosteroid may be used. [Refer to BNF 6.3.2 (glucocorticoid therapy).]

2.12 Answer B
Maculopapular rashes occur commonly in ampicillin treatment and are associated in patients with glandular fever. [Refer to BNF 5.1.1.3 (broad-spectrum penicillins).]

2.13 Answer E
Common side-effects associated with high-dose digoxin include anorexia, nausea, vomiting, diarrhoea, abdominal pain, visual disturbances, headache, fatigue and drowsiness.

2.14 Answer B
Patients using combined hormonal contraceptives should report any increase in headache frequency or onset of focal symptoms. [Refer to BNF 7.3.1 (oral contraceptives).] Other drugs on the list are used in the treatment or prophylaxis of migraine. [Refer to BNF 4.7.4 (anti-migraine drugs).]

2.15 Answer B
The sublingual route provides rapid relief of angina symptoms. [Refer to BNF 2.6.1 (nitrates).]

2.16 Answer A
Absorption of some oral antibacterials is increased or decreased by the presence of food and acid in the stomach. [Refer to BNF Appendix 9 (cautionary and advisory labels for dispensed products).]

2.17 Answer B
Tricyclic antidepressants may cause the following side-effects: antimuscarinic activity, blurred vision, constipation, drowsiness, sweating and urinary retention. [Refer to BNF 4.3.1 (tricyclic and related antidepressant drugs).]

2.18 **Answer D**

Women planning a pregnancy are advised to have an intake of folic acid at a dose of 400 micrograms daily before conception and during the first 12 weeks of pregnancy. [Refer to BNF 9.1.2 (drugs used in megaloblastic anaemia).]

2.19 **Answer B**

Hypokalaemia may result from thiazide treatment.

2.20 **Answer E**

Reduction in absorption due to tetracycline chelating polyvalent metal ions. [Refer to BNF Appendix 9 (cautionary and advisory labels for dispensed products).]

2.21 **Answer D**

Rifamycins induce hepatic enzyme activity and accelerate metabolism of oestrogens and progestogens, which may result in reduced effectiveness of both combined and progestogen-only oral contraceptives. [Refer to BNF 7.3.1 (combined hormonal contraceptives).]

2.22 **Answer A**

Amiodarone has the possibility to produce phototoxic reactions. The skin should be protected from light and a wide-spectrum sunscreen applied to safeguard against long ultraviolet and visible light. [Refer to BNF 2.3.2 (drugs for arrhythmias).]

2.23 **Answer C**

Foods and drinks containing amines should be avoided by patients taking monoamine-oxidase inhibitors (MAOIs) because of the risk of hypertensive crisis. [Refer to BNF 4.3.2 (monoamine-oxidase inhibitors).]

STYLE 2 – CLASSIFICATION TYPE

2.24 **Answer D**

Rifampicin induces microsomal enzyme activity. Reduced serum levels of a (second) given drug results from accelerated metabolism if it is metabolised by the same range of hepatic enzymes.

2.25 **Answer D**

Body secretions, such as urine and saliva, are coloured orange-red by rifampicin treatment.

2.26 **Answer A**

Quinolones may induce convulsions in those with a history of epilepsy or a predisposition to seizures. [Refer to BNF 5.1.12 (quinolones).]

2.27 **Answer C**

Oral nystatin is not systemically absorbed and has an indication for the treatment of *Candida* infections of the skin and mucous membranes, including intestinal candidiasis. [Refer to BNF 5.2 (antifungal drugs).]

2.28 **Answer E**

Reduced absorption of tetracyclines results from the formation of chelates if taken at the same time as milk, indigestion preparations, iron and zinc. Doxycycline, lymecycline and monocycline are less liable to form chelates with milk. [Refer to BNF Appendix 9 (cautionary and advisory labels for dispensed medicines).]

2.29 **Answer E**

Thiazolidinediones lower blood glucose levels by reducing peripheral insulin resistance. [Refer to BNF 6.1.2.3 (other antidiabetics).]

2.30 **Answer A**

Acarbose is an intestinal alpha glucosidase inhibitor, thereby delaying the digestion and absorption of starch and sucrose in the small intestine. [Refer to BNF 6.1.2.3 (other antidiabetics).]

2.31 **Answer D**

A side-effect of metformin is weight loss. Hence, this drug is an option in overweight patients with type 2 diabetes where strict dieting has not controlled the condition. [Refer to BNF 6.1.2.2 (biguanides).]

2.32 **Answer A**

Thiazides may aggravate diabetes.

2.33 **Answer E**

ACE inhibitors can cause renal impairment and should be avoided in patients with known or suspected renovascular disease, except in cases where blood pressure cannot be controlled by alternative medication. [Refer to BNF 2.5.5.1 (angiotensin-converting enzyme inhibitors).]

2.34 **Answer D**

Typical antipsychotic drugs are often associated with extrapyramidal symptoms. [Refer to BNF 4.2.1 (antipsychotic drugs).]

2.35 **Answer: D**

Phenytoin exhibits a narrow therapeutic index and a non-linear relationship between dose and plasma concentrations. Small dosage increases may result in large rises in plasma concentrations, leading to toxic side-effects. [Refer to BNF 4.8.1 (control of epilepsy).]

2.36 **Answer D**

Plasma concentrations of phenytoin are increased by voriconazole. [Refer to BNF Appendix 1 (interactions).]

2.37 **Answer A**

Amoxicillin is a broad-spectrum penicillin and is active against Gram-positive and Gram-negative bacteria. [Refer to 5.1.1.3 (broad-spectrum penicillins).]

2.38 **Answer C**

Erythromycin has an antibacterial spectrum similar to that of penicillin, and is an alternative in penicillin-allergic patients. [Refer to BNF 5.1.5 (macrolides).]

2.39 Answer E
Oral vancomycin does not have significant systemic absorption; it is used in the treatment of antibiotic-associated (pseudomembranous) colitis. [Refer to BNF 5.1.7 (some other antibacterials).]

2.40 Answer C
Finasteride is an anti-androgen, and has marketing authorisation (licensed) for use in benign prostatic hyperplasia and male-pattern baldness in men.

2.41 Answer D
Dosing intervals of methotrexate are at weekly intervals.

2.42 Answer A
Plasma concentrations of digoxin are increased by amiodarone. [Refer to BNF Appendix 1 (interactions).]

2.43 Answer B
The occurrence of hypokalaemia, with the use of diuretics, may increase the cardiac toxic effects of digoxin. [Refer to BNF Appendix 1 (interactions).]

2.44 Answer C
Colestyramine binds and reduces the absorption of digoxin.

See Chapter 1 for key to responses for this section

2.45 Answer E
HRT may be used for the prophylaxis of postmenopausal osteoporosis if initiated in the early stages of menopause and continued for up to 5 years. [Refer to BNF 6.6 (drugs affecting bone metabolism).] However, HRT may increase the risk of breast cancer, endometrial cancer and venous thromboembolism. [Refer to BNF 6.4.1.1 (oestrogens and HRT).]

2.46 Answer A
NSAIDs, colchicines and allopurinol are used in different stages of gout. [Refer to 10.1.4 (gout and cytotoxic-induced hyperuricaemia).]

2.47 Answer E
Colchicine and high-dose NSAIDs are oral treatments used in acute attacks of gout. [Refer to 10.1.4 (gout and cytotoxic-induced hyperuricaemia).]

2.48 Answer A
Different proprietary preparations of certain drugs may vary in bioavailability. It is best to avoid changing the formulation in order to prevent a reduced effect or excessive side-effects, i.e. prescriptions should specify brand of drug.

2.49 Answer B
The effectiveness of oral contraceptives may be reduced in the presence of drugs that induce hepatic enzyme activity and during the first 3 weeks of treatment with some broad-spectrum antibiotics. [Refer to BNF 7.3.1 (combined hormonal contraceptives).]

2.50 Answer B
Moderate amounts of alcohol may be consumed; the anticoagulant effect of warfarin may be increased if alcohol is consumed in large amounts. [Refer to BNF Appendix 1 (interactions).]

2.51 **Answer D**

Lithium withdrawal is required if there is evidence of overdose. Symptoms of lithium toxicity include: blurred vision, muscle weakness, increasing gastrointestinal disturbance (anorexia, vomiting, diarrhoea) and increased CNS disturbances (mild drowsiness, lack of co-ordination, coarse tremor).

2.52 **Answer B**

Potentially hazardous interaction if alcohol is taken with disulfiram or a tricyclic antidepressant. [Refer to BNF Appendix 1 (interactions).]

2.53 **Answer A**

Hepatic first-pass metabolism is prevented using formulations that avoid absorption in the gastrointestinal tract. Hence, the drug is delivered directly to the site of action or blood stream.

2.54 **Answer C**

Lipid-soluble drugs are able to enter and accumulate more readily in cells, resulting in a high volume of distribution compared to non-lipid-soluble drugs. In addition, highly lipid-soluble molecules are reabsorbed in the renal tubule by passive diffusion, preventing their excretion by the kidneys.

2.55 **Answer B**

Antifungals and calcium channel blockers increase the plasma concentration of theophylline, whereas tobacco is likely to decrease it. [Refer to BNF 3.1.3 (theophylline).]

2.56 **Answer C**

The metabolism of theophylline is inhibited by cimetidine, resulting in higher plasma levels and symptoms of theophylline overdose. [Refer to BNF 3.1.3 (theophylline).]

2.57 **Answer A**

Spacer devices, dry powder inhalers, and breath-actuated inhalers do not require co-ordination between actuation of a pressured metered-dose inhaler and inhalation. [Refer to BNF 3.1.5 (peak flow meters, inhaler devices and nebulisers).]

2.58 **Answer A**

Large-volume intravenous infusions should be isotonic and free from visible particles and preservatives.

2.59 **Answer B**

Candidates should be aware of the appropriate use and hazardous effects of medicines.

2.60 **Answer A**

NSAIDs have anti-inflammatory, analgesic and anti-pyretic properties. [Refer to BNF 10.1.1 (non-steroidal anti-inflammatory drugs).]

See Chapter 1 for key to responses for this section

2.61 **Answer C**
There is decreased production of clotting factors by the liver in patients with severe liver disease; oral anticoagulants are not advisable in such patients.

2.62 **Answer A**
Serum lithium concentrations can increase in the presence of thiazide diuretics; lithium excretion is reduced due to sodium depletion. [Refer to BNF 4.2.3 (antimanic drugs).]

2.63 **Answer A**
Abrupt withdrawal of phenobarbital may cause rebound seizures. [Refer to 4.8.1 (control of epilepsy).]

2.64 **Answer A**
Diabetic ketoacidosis is treated using soluble insulin by intravenous infusion or intramuscular injection. The absorption of insulin from subcutaneous injection may be slow and erratic. [Refer to BNF 6.1.3 (diabetic ketoacidosis).]

2.65 **Answer B**
Co-trimoxazole is contraindicated in the last trimester of pregnancy due to the risk of developing neonatal blood disorders. Trimethoprim has an anti-folate effect in the first trimester and poses a teratogenic risk. [Refer to BNF Appendix 4 (pregnancy).]

2.66 **Answer E**
Insulin requirements are increased when the body is under stress. [Refer to BNF 6.1.1 (insulins).]

2.67 **Answer D**
The pressor effect of tyramine, in some foods, may be potentiated if MAOIs remain in the body's circulation. [Refer to BNF 4.3.2 (monoamine-oxidase inhibitors).]

2.68 **Answer A**

Nystatin may be used to treat oral fungal infections as it is not absorbed from the gastrointestinal tract. [Refer to BNF 12.3.2 (oropharyngeal anti-infective drugs).] Nystatin cream and pessaries provide local treatment of vaginal infections. [Refer to BNF 7.2.2 (anti-infective drugs).]

2.69 **Answer C**

Diuretics may enhance the profound hypotensive effect that can result from starting ACE inhibitors. The combination of potassium-sparing diuretics and ACE inhibitors increases the risk of developing hyperkalaemia. [Refer to BNF 2.5.5.1 (angiotensin-converting enzyme inhibitors).]

2.70 **Answer B**

Aspirin increases the risk of bleeding, in patients taking warfarin, due to the nature of its antiplatelet effect. [Refer to BNF Appendix 1 (interactions).]

2 *Clinical pharmacy and therapeutics:* Open book

Section I   *20 answers*

2.71 **Answer C**

The ideal body-weight for a 3-year-old child is 15 kg, and prophylactic trimethoprim in children is 1–2 mg/kg at night; thus 30 mg trimethoprim is given. [Refer to BNF Prescribing for children (table detailing ideal body-weight and body surface for children of different ages).]

2.72 **Answer D**

Loop and thiazide diuretics antagonise the hypoglycaemic effect of antidiabetics. [Refer to BNF Appendix 1 (interactions).]

2.73 **Answer D**

Grapefruit juice increases the plasma concentration of dihydropyridine calcium-channel blockers (e.g. amlodipine, felodipine, nifedipine). [Refer to BNF Appendix 1 (interactions).]

2.74 **Answer E**

Use of tetracyclines should be avoided in mild renal impairment. [Refer to BNF Appendix 3 (renal impairment).]

2.75 **Answer E**

Patients with a prosthetic valve, or a history of endocarditis, who require dental surgery under general anaesthesia may, if they have a penicillin allergy, use the following antibiotics: vancomycin and gentamicin, teicoplanin and gentamicin, or clindamycin. [Refer to BNF 5.1 (antibacterial drugs).]

2.76 **Answer D**

Lifestyle changes and monthly blood pressure readings are recommended in those who have blood pressures of systolic 140–159 mmHg or diastolic 90–99 mmHg and no other complications. [Refer to BNF 2.5 (drugs affecting the renin-angiotensin system and some other antihypertensive drugs).]

2.77 **Answer C**

For most patients, a plasma theophylline concentration of 10–20 mg/litre is required for adequate bronchodilation. [Refer to BNF 3.1.1 (theophylline).]

2.78 **Answer D**

The main side-effects of theophylline are tachycardia, palpitations, nausea, headache, insomnia, arrhythmias and convulsions. [Refer to BNF 3.1.1 (theophylline).]

2.79 **Answer E**

Plasma theophylline concentrations are reduced by smoking, alcohol and by drugs that induce the activity of liver enzymes. Hence, a reduction in any of these factors may cause a rise in the blood levels of theophylline. [Refer to BNF 3.1.1 (theophylline).]

2.80 **Answer A**

AmBisome® (liposomal amphotericin) should be reconstituted with water for injections, and the resultant solution is introduced into glucose 5% infusion with a pH of not less than 4.2. [Refer to BNF Appendix 6 (intravenous additives).]

2.81 **Answer C**

A 5-HT$_1$ agonist is appropriate for treating an acute migraine attack when simple analgesics are ineffective. The other drugs mentioned are for prophylaxis, chronic recurrent attacks or only for hospital use. [Refer to BNF 4.7.4.1 (treatment of the acute migraine attack).]

2.82 **Answer B**

A maximum of four ergotamine 2 mg suppositories may be used in 1 week. [Refer to BNF 4.7.4.1 (treatment of the acute migraine attack).]

2.83 **Answer B**

Rashes almost always occur in patients with glandular fever taking ampicillin. [Refer to BNF 5.1.1.3 (broad-spectrum penicillins).]

2.84 Answer A
Side-effects of beta-blockers include bradycardia, heart failure, hypotension, conduction disorders, peripheral vasoconstriction, GI disturbance, fatigue and sleep disturbance.

2.85 Answer C
Small dosage increases in phenytoin in some patients may produce large rises in plasma concentrations with toxic side-effects. [Refer to BNF 4.8.1 (control of epilepsy).]

2.86 Answer A
Side-effects of beta$_2$-agonists include: fine tremor, nervous tension, headache, peripheral dilatation and palpitations. [Refer to BNF 2.1.1.1 (selective beta$_2$ agonists).]

2.87 Answer D
Fluoride supplements are not recommended when drinking water contains fluoride levels of greater than 700 micrograms/litre (0.7 parts per million). [Refer to BNF 9.5.3 (fluoride).]

2.88 Answer C
Oral anticoagulants are used in patients with mechanical prosthetic heart valves to prevent the development of emboli. An antiplatelet drug may be used as an adjunct to oral anticoagulants. [Refer to BNF 2.8.2 (oral anticoagulants).]

2.89 Answer C
Sodium chloride 0.9% solution contains 0.9 g, 150 mmol each of sodium and chloride ions.

2.90 Answer B
Aspirin does not have an indication for gout. [Refer to BNF 10.1.4 (gout and cytotoxic-induced hyperuricaemia).]

STYLE 2 – CLASSIFICATION TYPE

2.91 Answer D
Metformin is the drug of choice in overweight patients for whom dieting has failed to control diabetes. [Refer to BNF 6.1.2.2 (biguanides).]

2.92 Answer D
Metformin can provoke lactic acidosis, especially if the patient has renal impairment. [Refer to BNF 6.1.2.2 (biguanides).]

2.93 Answer A
Elderly patients are prone to the hazards of hypoglycaemia when a long-acting sulphonylurea is used. [Refer to BNF 6.1.2.1 (sulphonylureas).]

2.94 Answer D
Potassium-sparing diuretics are not contraindicated in liver failure.

2.95 Answer D
Potassium-sparing diuretics cause the retention of potassium; therefore, hyperkalaemia is a possible side-effect. [Refer to BNF 2.2.3 (potassium-sparing diuretics).]

2.96 Answer A
Thiazides inhibit sodium re-absorption at the beginning of the distal convoluted tubule. [Refer to BNF 2.2.1 (thiazides and related diuretics).]

2.97 Answer A
Quinolones should not be used in children. [Refer to BNF 5.1.12 (quinolones).]

2.98 Answer A
Ciprofloxacin can be used to treat gonorrhoea. [Refer to BNF 5.1.12 (quinolones).]

2.99 Answer E
Rifampicin can colour urine, saliva and other body secretions orange-red.

2.100 **Answer B**

Clindamycin should be discontinued immediately if diarrhoea develops, as this may be indicative of antibiotic-associated colitis. [Refer to BNF 5.1.6 (clindamycin).]

2.101 **Answer C**

Aminoglycosides are not absorbed from the gastrointestinal tract and must be given by injection for systemic infections. [Refer to BNF 5.1.4 (aminoglycosides).]

2.102 **Answer B**

Ciprofloxacin (or erythromycin) is used to treat *Campylobacter* enteritis infections. [Refer to BNF 5.1 (antibacterial drugs).]

2.103 **Answer E**

The use of nitrofurantoin is to be avoided in renal impairment. [Refer to BNF Appendix 3 (renal impairment).]

2.104 **Answer E**

Acebutolol, metoprolol, propranolol and timolol have a protective value against myocardial infarction, when started in the early convalescent phase. [Refer to BNF 2.4 (beta-adrenoceptor blocker drugs).]

2.105 **Answer A**

Bisoprolol and carvediol reduce mortality in stable heart failure. [Refer to BNF 2.4 (beta-adrenoceptor blocker drugs).]

STYLE 3 – MULTIPLE COMPLETION TYPE

See Chapter 1 for key to responses to this section

2.106 **Answer A**
Isotretinoin is better absorbed in the presence of food. Women should avoid wax epilation and dermabrasion for at least 6 months after stopping treatment. Furthermore, women of child-bearing age should practise effective contraception as isotretinoin is teratogenic. [Refer to BNF 13.6.2 (oral preparations for acne).]

2.107 **Answer E**
Manufacturers advise against the use of aspirin and NSAIDs during pregnancy, labour and delivery. [Refer to BNF Appendix 4 (pregnancy).]

2.108 **Answer A**
[Refer to BNF Appendix 3 (renal impairment).]

2.109 **Answer E**
Streptomycin is to be given intramuscularly. [Refer to BNF 5.1.9 (antituberculous drugs).]

2.110 **Answer D**
Arrhythmias is a possible sign of overdose, especially for the following: tricyclic antidepressants, some antipsychotics, some antihistamines and co-proxamol. [Refer to BNF 'Emergency treatment of poisoning'.]

2.111 **Answer D**
Metabolism of Nuelin SA® (theophylline) is inhibited by erythromycin (with decreased plasma-erythromycin concentration) and ciprofloxacin. [Refer to BNF 1 (interactions).]

2.112 **Answer C**
Side-effects of nifedipine include headache, flushing, dizziness, tachycardia, palpitations, gravitational oedema, rash, urticaria, nausea, constipation and diarrhoea.

2.113 **Answer C**

Digoxin side-effects, given as an overdose, include anorexia, nausea, vomiting, diarrhoea, abdominal pain, visual disturbance, headache, fatigue, drowsiness, confusion and arrhythmias. [Refer to BNF 2.1.1 (cardiac glycosides).]

2.114 **Answer A**

Inhibition of theophylline metabolism, resulting in increased plasma levels, may be caused by: beta blockers, cimetidine, ciprofloxacin, erythromycin, oral contraceptives and verapamil. [Refer to BNF Appendix 1 (interactions).]

2.115 **Answer B**

Ciprofloxacin or erythromycin is used to treat *Campylobacter* enteritis infections. [Refer to BNF 5.1 (antibacterial drugs).]

2.116 **Answer E**

Nitrofurantoin is to be avoided in renal impairment owing to the risk of peripheral neuropathy, and drug action is ineffective owing to inadequate urine concentrations. [Refer to BNF Appendix 3 (renal impairment).]

2.117 **Answer B**

The main risk of a paracetamol overdose is liver damage due to the production of *N*-acetylbenzoquinoneimine (a toxic quinone intermediate). Treatment options include preventing the absorption of paracetamol in the gastrointestinal tract (using activated charcoal), and antidotes to protect the liver (acetylcysteine, methionine). [Refer to BNF 'Emergency treatment of poisoning'.]

2.118 **Answer D**

Blood dyscrasia is a side-effect of carbamazepine and sodium valproate; increased risk of developing blood dyscrasia if both drugs are taken together. Concurrent use is not contraindicated but there should be appropriate monitoring of serum levels. [Refer to BNF 4.8.1 (control of epilepsy).]

2.119 **Answer A**

[Refer to BNF Appendix 2 (liver disease).]

2.120 **Answer C**
[Refer to BNF 3.1.1.1 (selective beta$_2$ agonists).]

2.121 **Answer A**
[Refer to BNF Appendix 1 (interactions).]

2.122 **Answer A**

See Chapter 1 for key to responses for this section

2.123 Answer D
Caution is needed when a diuretic is taken with a cardiac glycoside as hypokalaemia predisposes to digitalis toxicity. [Refer to BNF 2.1.1 (cardiac glycosides).]

2.124 Answer C
Peak serum concentrations, taken at 1-hour post-dose, should be 5–10 mg/litre (3–5 mg/litre for streptococcal or enterococcal endocarditis); pre-dose (trough) concentration should be less than 2 mg/litre (less than 1 mg/litre for streptococcal or enterococcal endocarditis). [Refer to BNF 5.1.4 (aminoglycosides).]

2.125 Answer A
The main side-effects of aminoglycosides are nephrotoxicity and ototoxicity. If the pre-dose serum concentrations are high the interval between doses must be increased. [Refer to BNF 5.1.4 (aminoglycosides).]

2.126 Answer A
Use of Phosex® tablets suggests that the patient is in renal failure. Gliquidone is to be avoided in such situations.

2.127 Answer E
ACE inhibitors should be given to all diabetics with nephropathy causing proteinuria or with established microalbuminuria, provided that there are no contraindications. This therapy may potentiate the hypoglycaemic effect of insulin and oral antidiabetic drugs. [Refer to BNF 6.1.5 (treatment of diabetic nephropathy and neuropathy).]

2.128 Answer C
Triazole antifungals increase plasma concentration of sulphonylureas. [Refer to BNF Appendix 1 (interactions).]

2.129 **Answer C**

Plasma concentration of digoxin is increased by nifedipine (Tensipine MR®), and hypokalaemia (resulting from diuretics) predisposes to digitalis toxicity. [Refer to BNF Appendix 1 (interactions).]

2.130 **Answer E**

Crystal violet is not recommended for application to mucous membranes or open wounds.

2.131 **Answer A**

Oral progestogen-only contraceptives should be taken at the same time each day; if delayed by longer than three hours contraceptive protection may be lost. [Refer to BNF 7.3.2.1 (oral progestogen-only contraceptives).]

2.132 **Answer C**

Each Solpadol preparation contains 500 mg of paracetamol, which has a maximum daily dose of 4 g.

3 *Pharmacy practice:* closed book

Section I   *17 answers*

3.1 **Answer A**
Categories of evidence include:
Level 1: randomised control trials
Level 2: controlled studies without randomisation
Level 3: descriptive studies (i.e. comparative studies,
        correlation studies and case–control studies)
Level 4: expert opinion

3.2 **Answer C**
Suspected adverse reactions for the following should be
reported to the Committee of Safety of Medicines, and
Medicines and Healthcare products Regulatory Agency:

- new drugs and vaccines (indicated by inverted black
  triangle symbol ▼)

- any therapeutic agent, including herbal medicines

- all serious adverse reactions for established medicines

- all suspected reactions in children

- delayed drug effects

- congenital abnormalities

[Refer to BNF adverse reaction to drugs.]

3.3 **Answer E**
Concentrated chloroform water BP requires dilution of 1 in 40
to produce chloroform water BP.

3.4 **Answer D**
Clinical governance makes NHS organisations accountable for
improving services and safeguarding high standards of care.

3.5 **Answer A**
Audit can occur in any aspect of pharmacy practice. It
determines the level of service against a set of objectives.
Audits and patient questionnaires are not mandatory in
pharmacy practice.

3.6 **Answer C**

Glyceryl trinitrate tablets are supplied in a glass container with a foil-lined cap and no cotton wool wadding. The container must not hold more than 100 tablets, which should be discarded after 8 weeks from opening.

3.7 **Answer A**

Aspirin degradation occurs mainly from hydrolysis.

3.8 **Answer C**

The use of preservatives is to prevent microbial contamination during use.

3.9 **Answer E**

Inhaled corticosteroids are used as prophylactic treatment of asthma, and thus require regular use. A steroid card is given to patients on high doses. Oral candidiasis is reduced by rinsing the mouth with water after using the inhaler. [Refer to BNF 3.2 (corticosteroids).]

3.10 **Answer B**

Glyceryl trinitrate tablets are taken sublingually for the prophylaxis and treatment of angina.

3.11 **Answer D**

Refrigerators are used for products requiring storage at temperatures between 2 and 8°C.

3.12 **Answer A**

Endorsing prescriptions for Schedule 2 or 3 controlled drugs attracts additional professional fees. [Refer to Drug Tariff Part IIIA (professional fees).]

3.13 **Answer D**

The role of the Medicines and Healthcare products Regulatory Agency is to ensure acceptable standards of quality, safety and efficacy for drugs and devices used for therapeutic purposes.

3.14 **Answer D**

Eye drops, supplied in multiple application containers, should be discarded 28 days after opening (7 days in hospital setting). [Refer to BNF 11.2 (control of microbial contamination).]

3.15 **Answer C**
'Store in cool place' requires a storage temperature between 8 and 15°C.

3.16 **Answer A**
The prescriber should be contacted as bioavailability of Adalat® (nifedipine) capsules and modified-release tablets varies. The patient should be told about the problem in a manner that does not undermine their confidence in the prescriber.

3.17 **Answer E**
Glyceryl trinitrate tablets should be discarded 8 weeks after opening the container.

STYLE 2 – CLASSIFICATION TYPE

3.18 Answer E
[Refer to Medicine, Ethics and Practice: a Guide for Pharmacists 1.3 (alphabetical list of medicines for human use).]

3.19 Answer E
[Refer to Medicine, Ethics and Practice: a Guide for Pharmacists 1.2.11 (controlled drugs).]

3.20 Answer A
[Refer to 'Medicines information services' and 'Index of manufacturers'.]

3.21 Answer C
Products to be sold in the UK will display their 'Marketing Authorisation' on the packaging.

3.22 Answer A
Suspected adverse drug reactions are the yellow forms in the BNF.

3.23 Answer B
[Refer to Drug Tariff Part VIA (payment for additional professional fees).]

3.24 Answer B
[Refer to Drug Tariff Part XVI (notes on charges).]

3.25 Answer D
Dilsulfiram-like reaction occurs when metronidazole is taken with alcohol. [Refer to BNF Appendix 9 (cautionary and advisory labels for dispensed medicines).]

3.26 Answer B
Rifampicin must be taken over long periods; the patient may believe that they are not deriving benefit from the treatment. [Refer to BNF Appendix 9 (cautionary and advisory labels for dispensed medicines).]

See Chapter 1 for key to responses for this section

3.27 Answer D
Research requires approval by an ethics committee, and
notification to the Data Protection Commissioner is required
if a person can be identified from the collected information.
Audits do not necessarily require ethics committee approval
or registration under the Data Protection Act 1998. However,
appropriate members of staff should be informed when an
audit is being conducted.

3.28 Answer D
National Service Frameworks define national standards and
models for a particular service or patient group.

3.29 Answer C
Glyceryl trinitrate sublingual tablets are placed under the
tongue and allowed to dissolve. They are discarded 8 weeks
after the container is opened.

3.30 Answer B
Theophylline has a narrow therapeutic window and
bioavailability differs between brands. A prescription for
theophylline should specify the brand to be dispensed
[Refer to BNF 3.1.3 (theophylline).] Beta-blockers are not
recommended in asthmatics, unless there is no alternative,
due to the risk of provoking bronchospasm. [Refer to BNF
3.1.3 (theophylline).]

3.31 Answer A
[Refer to Medicine, Ethics and Practice: a Guide for
Pharmacists 3.3.1 (clinical governance).]

3.32 Answer C
The item stated on NHS prescriptions must be dispensed,
including brand-specific medicines. This does not apply to
products that are listed in the Drug Tariff Part XVIIIA (drugs
and other substances not to be prescribed under the NHS
Pharmaceutical Services).

3.33 **Answer D**

The National Institute for Clinical Excellence is tasked to develop clinical guidelines, evaluate health technology and authoritative clinical guidance for the NHS in England and Wales.

3.34 **Answer B**

Appropriate risk management procedures should operate in pharmacies. [Refer to Medicine, Ethics and Practice: a Guide for Pharmacists 3.2 (guidance on good practice).]

3.35 **Answer A**

Lifelong learning is a continual process of reviewing and updating knowledge and skills that are relevant to professional practice. [Refer to Medicine, Ethics and Practice: a Guide for Pharmacists 3.3.2 (continuing professional practice).]

3.36 **Answer E**

An audit is a process involving the evaluation of professional service against a set of standards.

3.37 **Answer B**

Sources of drug information should be evidence-based.

3.38 **Answer A**

Plastic materials can absorb constituents of a medicinal product, such as antimicrobial preservatives and stabilising agents. This may lead to decreased stability of the product and reduced shelf-life.

3.39 **Answer E**

Newly licensed medicines are identified by the inverted black triangle symbol ▼.

3.40 Answer A

Suspected adverse reactions for the following should be reported to the Committee of Safety of Medicines, and Medicines and Healthcare products Regulatory Agency:

- new drugs and vaccines (indicated by inverted black triangle symbol ▼)
- any therapeutic agent, including herbal medicines
- all serious adverse reactions for established medicines
- all suspected reactions in children
- delayed drug effects
- congenital abnormalities

[Refer to BNF adverse reaction to drugs.]

3.41 Answer B

Sterile products need to be manufactured in conditions that minimise the risks of contamination from microbes, particulates and pyrogens; protective clothing must be worn to achieve this objective.

3.42 Answer E

Insulin injections are available as solutions (short-acting), suspensions (intermediate/long-acting), and as a suspension in solution (biphasic). They should be stored in a refrigerator and not allowed to freeze. All injections should be sterile and pyrogen-free.

3.43 Answer A

Breath-actuated inhalers, dry-powder inhalers and spacer devices are used to assist patients with poor inhaler technique. [Refer to BNF 3.1.5 (peak flow meters, inhaler devices and nebulisers).]

3.44 Answer A

Vaccines should be stored away from light, not be allowed to freeze, and most will need to be kept between 2 and 8°C. [Refer to BNF 14.3 (storage and use).]

3.45 Answer A

[Refer to Medicine, Ethics and Practice: a Guide for Pharmacists 3 (service specifications).]

STYLE 4 – ASSERTION–REASON TYPE

See Chapter 1 for key to responses for this section

3.46 Answer D

Medicines returned to the pharmacy from a patient or carer must be appropriately disposed off and not returned to stock. [Refer to Medicine, Ethics and Practice: a Guide for Pharmacists 3 (service specifications).]

3.47 Answer A

The Cochrane Collaboration prepares, maintains and promotes the accessibility of systematic reviews relating to healthcare interventions.

3.48 Answer D

[Refer to Medicine, Ethics and Practice: a Guide for Pharmacists 1.2.6 (labelling of medicinal products).]

3.49 Answer C

Disulfiram-like adverse reaction, resulting from taking metronidazole and alcohol, is not related to impaired absorption of either drug.

3.50 Answer A

A terminal sterilisation process should be used wherever possible for the manufacture of aqueous products under aseptic conditions.

3.51 Answer A

Most vaccines should be stored in a refrigerator, protected from sunlight, and not be allowed to freeze. [Refer to BNF 14.3 (storage and use).]

3.52 Answer A

Oil-based preparations can damage condoms and contraceptive diaphragms made from latex rubber. [Refer to BNF 7.3.3 (spermicidal contraceptives).]

3 *Pharmacy practice:* Open book

Section I   *13 answers*

3.53 **Answer E**

[Refer to Drug Tariff Part XVI (notes on charges).]

3.54 **Answer D**

Analog XP® has been approved by the Advisory Committee on Borderline Substances for use in patients with phenylketonuria. [Refer to BNF Appendix 7 (borderline substances) or Drug Tariff XV (borderline substances).]

3.55 **Answer C**

Different formulations of the same medicinal component attract a separate NHS prescription charge. However, if the formulation is the same but two different strengths of the preparation are required this would attract only one charge. [Refer to Drug Tariff Part XVI (notes on charges).]

3.56 **Answer E**

Newly licensed medicines are identified by the inverted black triangle symbol ▼.

3.57 **Answer E**

Nepro® liquid has been approved by the Advisory Committee on Borderline Substances for use in patients in renal failure. [Refer to BNF Appendix 7 (borderline substances) or Drug Tariff XV (borderline substances).]

3.58 **Answer D**

[Refer to Drug Tariff Part XVI (notes on charges).]

3.59 **Answer A**

Doctors, pharmacists and nurses can initiate reports on suspected adverse reactions. The following should be reported to the Committee of Safety of Medicines, and Medicines and Healthcare products Regulatory Agency:

- new drugs and vaccines (indicated by inverted black triangle symbol ▼)
- any therapeutic agent, including herbal medicines
- all serious adverse reactions for established medicines
- all suspected reactions in children
- delayed drug effects
- congenital abnormalities

[Refer to BNF adverse reaction to drugs.]

3.60 **Answer A**

Pharmacists will not be reimbursed by the Pricing Prescription Authority if they dispense an item which is 'blacklisted'. [Refer to Drug Tariff Part XVIIIA (drugs and other substances not to be prescribed under the NHS pharmaceutical services).]

3.61 **Answer B**

The MMR (measles, mumps and rubella) vaccine is routinely given as a single dose to infants between 12 and 15 months of age. [Refer to BNF 14.1 (active immunity).]

3.62 **Answer A**

[Refer to Drug Tariff Part XVI (notes on charges).]

3.63 **Answer E**

The following medicines are unsuitable for dispensing into monitored dosage systems: buccal tablets, dispersible tablets, effervescent tablets, sublingual tablets, hygroscopic preparations and cytotoxic preparations. [Refer to Medicine, Ethics and Practice: a Guide for Pharmacists 3.4.7 (monitored dosage system).]

3.64 **Answer D**

[Refer to Drug Tariff Part XVI (notes on charges).]

3.65 **Answer B**

100 g of aqueous cream BP contains 30 g of emulsifying ointment (i.e. 30%). [Refer to BNF monograph for aqueous cream BP.]

100 g of emulsifying ointment BP contains 30 g of emulsifying wax (i.e. 30%). [Refer to BNF monograph for emulsifying ointment BP.]

Calculation:

$\{30 \times 30/100\}\%$ = 0.9% w/w of emulsifying wax in aqueous cream BP

3.66 Answer A

Patients with epilepsy requiring continuous anti-convulsive therapy are exempt from prescription charges.

3.67 Answer C

Different preparations of the same medicinal component attract a separate NHS prescription charge.[Refer to Drug Tariff Part XVI (notes on charges).]

3.68 Answer B

If the formulation is the same but two different strengths of the preparation are required this would attract only one charge. [Refer to Drug Tariff Part XVI (notes on charges).]

3.69 Answer C

Different formulations of the same medicinal component attract a separate NHS prescription charge. [Refer to Drug Tariff Part XVI (notes on charges).]

3.70 Answer B

The same type of dressing but in two different sizes would attract only one charge. [Refer to Drug Tariff Part XVI (notes on charges).]

3.71 Answer A

No charge is payable for contraceptive products or contraceptive appliances listed in the drugs tariff. [Refer to Drug Tariff Part XVI (notes on charges).]

3.72 Answer D

Metronidazole is the first-line treatment for *Giardia lamblia* infections . [Refer to BNF 5.6.4 (antigiardial drugs).]

3.73 Answer E

Items not listed in the dental practitioners' formulary cannot be prescribed on an NHS dental prescription form. [Refer to BNF Dental Practitioners' Formulary or Drug Tariff Part XVIIA (dental prescribing).]

3.74 **Answer B**
Betnovate-C® ointment can stain clothing.

3.75 **Answer D**
Halcinonide is a very potent topical corticosteroid.

3.76 **Answer E**
Synalar N® cream contains hydroxybenzoates (parabens) which result in a sensitivity reaction in some patients. [Refer to BNF 13.1.3 (excipients and sensitisation).]

STYLE 3 – MULTIPLE COMPLETION TYPE

See Chapter 1 for key to responses for this section

3.77 **Answer A**
Suspected adverse reactions to medical devices should be
reported to the Medicine and Healthcare products Regulatory
Agency. [Refer to BNF Adverse reactions to drugs.]

3.78 **Answer D**
Cabergoline must be dispensed in the original container as a
desiccant is part of the packaging.

3.79 **Answer C**
Items not listed in the dental practitioners' formulary cannot
be prescribed on an NHS dental prescription form. [Refer
to BNF Dental Practitioners' Formulary or Drug Tariff Part
XVIIA (dental prescribing).]

3.80 **Answer A**
Blacklisted products are not to be prescribed on an NHS
prescription. [Refer to Drug Tariff Part XVIIIA (drugs
and other substances not to be prescribed under the NHS
pharmaceutical services).]

3.81 **Answer C**
Appliances listed in the Drug Tariff would be reimbursed by
the Prescription Pricing Authority. [Refer to Drug Tariff Part
IX (appliances).]

3.82 **Answer D**
Items not listed in the dental practitioners' formulary cannot
be prescribed on an NHS dental prescription form. [Refer
to BNF Dental Practitioners' Formulary or Drug Tariff Part
XVIIA (dental prescribing).]

3.83 **Answer A**

The following should be reported to the Committee of Safety of Medicines, and Medicines and Healthcare products Regulatory Agency:

- new drugs and vaccines (indicated by inverted black triangle symbol ▼)
- any therapeutic agent, including herbal medicines
- all serious adverse reactions for established medicines
- all suspected reactions in children
- delayed drug effects
- congenital abnormalities

[Refer to BNF adverse reaction to drugs.]

3.84 **Answer D**

[Refer to Drug Tariff Part XVI (notes on charges).]

3.85 **Answer B**

[Refer to Drug Tariff Part XVI (notes on charges).]

3.86 **Answer E**

Clobazam is used in the treatment of anxiety and epilepsy. It may be dispensed on an NHS prescription if the prescriber has endorsed 'SLS'. [Refer to Drug Tariff Part XVIIIB (drugs to be prescribed in certain circumstances under the NHS pharmaceutical services).]

3.87 **Answer A**

[Refer to BNF Appendix 9 (cautionary and advisory labels for dispensed medicines).]

3.88 **Answer A**

[Refer to Drug Tariff Part VIA (payment for additional professional services).]

See Chapter 1 for key to responses for this section

3.89 **Answer A**
Contraceptive devices and spermicidal preparations listed in the Drug Tariff may be prescribed on an NHS prescription form. [Refer to Drug Tariff Part IX (appliances).]

3.90 **Answer D**
Glyceryl trinitrate is not compatible with polyvinyl chloride infusion containers. [Refer to BNF Appendix 6 (intravenous additives).]

3.91 **Answer D**
Antacids can produce an alkaline (or less acidic) environment which may cause products with enteric coatings to undergo premature dissolution. [Refer to BNF Appendix 9 (cautionary and advisory labels for dispensed medicines).]

3.92 **Answer A**
Pharmacists providing domiciliary oxygen should monitor the progress of patients requiring this service and establish good communication channels with the patient's GP. [Refer to Medicine, Ethics and Practice: a Guide for Pharmacists 3.1.3 (practice guidance for pharmacists providing domiciliary oxygen services).]

3.93 **Answer A**
The Advisory Committee on Borderline Substances advises on the circumstances under which certain food products may be prescribed on an NHS prescription. [Refer to BNF Appendix 7 (borderline substances) or Drug Tariff Part XV (borderline substances).]

3.94 **Answer D**
The maximum dose of chloroquine for prophylaxis of malaria is 300 mg once weekly. [Refer to BNF 5.4.1 (antimalarials).]

4 *Pharmacy law and ethics:* Closed book

STYLE 1 – SIMPLE COMPLETION TYPE

4.1 **Answer B**

Pharmacy medicines which are liable to be misused include: preparations containing codeine, ephedrine, morphine, antihistamines; cyclizine; laxatives; antihistamines alone; sympathomimetics; and high-dose caffeine preparations. [Refer to Medicine, Ethics and Practice: a Guide for Pharmacists: substances of misuse.]

4.2 **Answer B**

The quantity of an emergency supply which is allowed to be dispensed at the request of a patient should be no greater than that which will provide 5 days' treatment; a full cycle of an oral contraceptive; and the smallest pack available for creams, insulin and inhalers. [Refer to Medicine, Ethics and Practice: a Guide for Pharmacists: emergency supplies of prescription-only medicines.]

4.3 **Answer C**

Pharmacists are required to interview the patient personally if a request for the emergency hormonal contraceptive is made. [Refer to Medicine, Ethics and Practice: a Guide for Pharmacists: the supply of emergency hormonal contraception as a pharmacy medicine.]

4.4 **Answer C**

Section 9 of the Medicines Act 1968, as amended, enables a practitioner to order a product that has no marketing authorisation to be used for their patient. The law also allows a pharmacist to dispense such a product in accordance with the requirements of the prescription.

4.5 **Answer E**

The options, based on the COSHH Regulations 1997, for preventing or controlling exposure to a hazardous substance are: (in order of the most preferred)

1 *elimination of the use of the substance*
2 *substitution with a less hazardous substance*
3 *substitution with a less hazardous form of the substance*
4 *handle the substance in an isolation cabinet*
5 *wear suitable personal protective equipment*

4.6 **Answer D**

[Refer to Medicine, Ethics and Practice: a Guide for Pharmacists: emergency supplies of prescription-only medicines.]

4.7 **Answer E**

Under the Data Protection Act 1998, if confidential information is to be kept then the Data Protection Commissioner must be notified. [Refer to Medicine, Ethics and Practice: a Guide for Pharmacists: patient medication records.]

4.8 **Answer E**

Medicines brought into hospital by the patient remain their own property. [Refer to Medicine, Ethics and Practice: a Guide for Pharmacists: medicines for hospital inpatients.]

4.9 **Answer E**

The main concern of a pharmacist is to act in the interests of patients and other members of the public. [Refer to Medicine, Ethics and Practice: a Guide for Pharmacists: key responsibilities of a pharmacist.]

4.10 **Answer E**

The Royal Pharmaceutical Society of Great Britain is not legally empowered to act as a trade union.

4.11 **Answer E**

There are 24 members of the Council of the Royal Pharmaceutical Society of Great Britain.

STYLE 2 – CLASSIFICATION TYPE

4.12 **Answer E**
[Refer to Medicine, Ethics and Practice: a Guide for
Pharmacists: alphabetical list of medicines for human use.]

4.13 **Answer E**
[Refer to Medicine, Ethics and Practice: a Guide for
Pharmacists: controlled drugs.]

4.14 **Answer A**
[Refer to 'Medicines information services' and 'Index of
manufacturers'.]

4.15 **Answer C**
Products to be sold in the UK will display their 'Marketing
Authorisation' on the packaging.

4.16 **Answer A**
Suspected adverse drug reactions are the yellow forms in the
BNF.

4.17 **Answer B**
[Refer to Drug Tariff Part VIA (payment for additional
professional fees).]

4.18 **Answer B**
[Refer to Drug Tariff Part XVI (notes on charges).]

Section III

See Chapter 1 for key to responses for this section

4.19 Answer E
The validity of prescriptions is shown in Table 7.1.

Table 7.1 Validity of prescriptions

Type of prescription	Validity from the date of issue
Non-repeat prescription	6 months
Repeat prescription	1st dispensing must be within 6 months
Schedule 2 or 3 controlled drugs	13 weeks

4.20 Answer E
[Refer to Medicine, Ethics and Practice: a Guide for Pharmacists: emergency supplies of prescription-only medicines.]

4.21 Answer D
Continuing professional development is used to reflect and identify personal learning needs. Continuing education courses are one means of meeting the learning needs. [Refer to Medicine, Ethics and Practice: a Guide for Pharmacists: continuing professional development.]

4.22 Answer A
[Refer to Medicine, Ethics and Practice: a Guide for Pharmacists: pharmacy premises and facilities.]

4.23 Answer A
Temazepam is a Schedule 3 controlled drug but is exempt from the handwriting requirements. [Refer to Medicine, Ethics and Practice: a Guide for Pharmacists: Schedule 3 drugs (CD no register).]

4.24 Answer C
Audit is a process that determines the level of service against a set of standards. [Refer to Medicine, Ethics and Practice: a Guide for Pharmacists: audit.]

4.25 Answer B
Pethidine is a Schedule 2 controlled drug. [Refer to Medicine, Ethics and Practice: a Guide for Pharmacists: Schedule 2 drugs (CD) and possession and supply of controlled drugs.]

4.26 Answer C
Prescription handwriting requirements apply to Schedule 2 and 3 controlled drugs. [Refer to Medicine, Ethics and Practice: a Guide for Pharmacists: prescription for controlled drugs.]

4.27 Answer B
The principles of clinical governance include:
1 identifiable persons that are accountable and responsible for the overall quality of care
2 quality improvement training
3 risk management policies
4 processes that identify and resolve poor performance
[Refer to Medicine, Ethics and Practice: a Guide for Pharmacists: service specification.]

4.28 Answer E
The keeping of patient medication records (PMR) requires notification to the Data Protection Commissioner. Patients may request disclosure of the information held on PMRs, but there is no immediate need to do so and the patient may have to pay a fee.

4.29 Answer B
The prescribing of Schedule 2 controlled drugs is restricted to medical practitioners who are registered with the General Medical Council. [Refer to Medicine, Ethics and Practice: a Guide for Pharmacists: prescriptions for controlled drugs.]

4.30 Answer A
The Health and Safety Act 1974 requires the following details to be entered in the accident book:
1 gender of the injured person
2 occupation of the injured person
3 nature of the injury
4 first aid given
5 any measure taken to prevent recurrence

4.31 **Answer E**

Diazepam is a Schedule 4 controlled drug and prescription handwriting requirements do not apply. [Refer to Medicine, Ethics and Practice: a Guide for Pharmacists: schedule 4 drugs.]

4.32 **Answer A**

The Health and Safety at Work Act 1974 includes the following:
1 maintenance of plant and systems of work
2 procedures for safe use, handling, storage and transport of articles and substances
3 training and supervision necessary to ensure health and safety of employees

4.33 **Answer E**

Unwanted medicines must be given to an assigned authority for the destruction of special waste. [Refer to Medicine, Ethics and Practice: a Guide for Pharmacists: collection and disposal of pharmaceutical waste.]

4.34 **Answer A**

Phenobarbital is a Schedule 3 controlled drug; it is subject to prescription handwriting requirements, as well as normal prescription requirements. [Refer to Medicine, Ethics and Practice: a Guide for Pharmacists: Schedule 3 drugs (CD no register).]

4.35 **Answer E**

The code of ethics provides guidance on the conduct of pharmacists, and may be applied to all pharmacists within and away from the practice of pharmacy. It is not a requirement of the Medicines Act 1968.

STYLE 4 – ASSERTION–REASON TYPE

See Chapter 1 for key to responses for this section

4.36 **Answer D**

It is permissible to use anonymised data for the purpose of research. [Refer to Medicine, Ethics and Practice: a Guide for Pharmacists: confidentiality.]

4.37 **Answer D**

The pharmacist must provide supervision when prescriptions are handed out, and during the sale and supply of medicines. It is a requirement of the Medicines Act 1968 that a registered pharmacy remains under the personal control of a pharmacist. Personal control is understood not to have ceased if the pharmacist is absent from the pharmacy for no longer than 30 minutes. [Refer to Medicine, Ethics and Practice: a Guide for Pharmacists: personal control.]

4.38 **Answer C**

The person most familiar with the procedure should write the standard operating procedure. [Refer to Medicine, Ethics and Practice: a Guide for Pharmacists: guidance on developing and implementing standard operating procedures for dispensing.]

4.39 **Answer A**

Possessing personal data requires notification to the Data Protection Commissioner. [Refer to Medicine, Ethics and Practice: a Guide for Pharmacists: patient medication records.]

4.40 **Answer A**

Pharmacists should be satisfied with the quality and source of medicines that they supply. [Refer to Medicine, Ethics and Practice: a Guide for Pharmacists: stock.]

4.41 **Answer B**

Emergency supplies at the request of a patient should only be carried out if there is an immediate need for the medication and the patient has been unable to get a new prescription for them. [Refer to Medicine, Ethics and Practice: a Guide for Pharmacists: emergency supplies of prescription-only medicines.]

4 *Pharmacy law and ethics:* Open book

Section I   *5 answers*

4.42 **Answer C**
[Refer to Medicine, Ethics and Practice: a Guide for
Pharmacists: pharmacy medicines (P).]

4.43 **Answer A**
Schedule 5 controlled drugs are not subject to the prescription
requirements of the Misuse of Drugs Regulations 2001 as
amended; hence emergency supplies may be allowed. [Refer
to Medicine, Ethics and Practice: a Guide for Pharmacists:
Schedule 5 drugs (CD inv).]

4.44 **Answer E**
Morphine sulphate oral solution 10 mg/5 ml is a Schedule
5 controlled drug and is not subject to safe custody
requirements. [Refer to Medicine, Ethics and Practice: a Guide
for Pharmacists: Schedule 5 drugs (CD inv).]

4.45 **Answer A**
Endorsing prescriptions for Schedule 2 or 3 controlled drugs
attracts additional professional fees. [Refer to Drug Tariff Part
IIIA (professional fees).]

4.46 **Answer C**
A medical practitioner may obtain up to 3 litres of industrial
methylated spirits on one signed order. [Refer to Medicine,
Ethics and Practice: a Guide for Pharmacists: IMS and DEB.]

Style 2 – Classification type

4.47 Answer C
Schedule 5 controlled drugs do not require a licence for import or export. [Refer to Medicine, Ethics and Practice: a Guide for Pharmacists: possession and supply of controlled drugs.]

4.48 Answer D
Schedule 2 and 3 controlled drugs have to meet controlled drug handwriting requirements. Temazepam and phenobarbital are exempt from this requirement. [Refer to Medicine, Ethics and Practice: a Guide for Pharmacists: prescriptions for controlled drugs.]

4.49 Answer E
Phenobarbital may be issued on an emergency supply basis provided it is only for the treatment of epilepsy. [Refer to Medicine, Ethics and Practice: a Guide for Pharmacists: emergency supplies of prescription-only medicines.]

4.50 Answer A
All Schedule 3 controlled drugs are exempt from safe custody requirements, except buprenorphine, diethylpropion, flunitrazepam and temazepam. [Refer to Medicine, Ethics and Practice: a Guide for Pharmacists: Schedule 3 drugs (CD no register).]

4.51 Answer E
Phenobarbital is exempt from the handwriting requirements of controlled drugs. [Refer to Medicine, Ethics and Practice: a Guide for Pharmacists: prescriptions for controlled drugs.]

4.52 Answer A
[Refer to Medicine, Ethics and Practice: a Guide for Pharmacists: alphabetical list of medicines for human use.]

4.53 Answer D
[Refer to Medicine, Ethics and Practice: a Guide for Pharmacists: alphabetical list of medicines for human use.]

Section III   *12 answers*

See Chapter 1 for key to responses for this section

4.54 Answer B
[Refer to Medicine, Ethics and Practice: a Guide for Pharmacists: guidance on writing SOPs.]

4.55 Answer C
[Refer to Medicine, Ethics and Practice: a Guide for Pharmacists: prescription-only veterinary drugs (POM) and labelling veterinary drugs.]

4.56 Answer C
[Refer to Medicine, Ethics and Practice: a Guide for Pharmacists: services to drug misusers.]

4.57 Answer E
[Refer to Medicine, Ethics and Practice: a Guide for Pharmacists: ambulance paramedics – administration.]

4.58 Answer C
If a child is deemed Gillick competent then they are legally recognised as being able to make an informed decision regarding their own medical treatment. As such, any information they disclose must remain confidential. [Refer to Medicine, Ethics and Practice: a Guide for Pharmacists: confidentiality.]

4.59 Answer C
[Refer to Medicine, Ethics and Practice: a Guide for Pharmacists: delivery services.]

4.60 Answer B
[Refer to Medicine, Ethics and Practice: a Guide for Pharmacists: paracetamol legal status.]

4.61 Answer A
[Refer to Medicine, Ethics and Practice: a Guide for Pharmacists: ophthalmic opticians – sale or supply.]

4.62 **Answer D**

The prime concern of a pharmacist is the welfare of the
patient and members of the public; hence, there is a duty to
report other pharmacists who may be considered a risk to
the safety of patients or the public. [Refer to Medicine, Ethics
and Practice: a Guide for Pharmacists: pharmacists providing
professional services.]

4.63 **Answer B**

Pharmacies should not sell products which may be considered
injurious to health or bring the pharmacy profession into
disrepute. [Refer to Medicine, Ethics and Practice: a Guide for
Pharmacists: stock.]

4.64 **Answer B**

[Refer to Medicine, Ethics and Practice: a Guide for
Pharmacists: chemicals.]

4.65 **Answer C**

[Refer to Medicine, Ethics and Practice: a Guide for
Pharmacists: labelling of relevant medicinal products.]

STYLE 4 – ASSERTION–REASON TYPE

See Chapter 1 for key to responses for this section

4.66 Answer D

Buprenorphine is a Schedule 3 controlled drug and cannot be dispensed as an emergency supply under any circumstances. [Refer to Medicine, Ethics and Practice: a Guide for Pharmacists: emergency supplies of prescription-only medicines.]

4.67 Answer B

Strychnine is classified as a Schedule 1 poison and has to fulfil the Pesticide Legislation which requires supply in the original manufacturer's packaging and in units of not more than 2 g. [Refer to Medicine, Ethics and Practice: a Guide for Pharmacists: alphabetical list of non-medicinal poisons.]

4.68 Answer D

A midwife is allowed to possess diamorphine, morphine, pethidine and pentazocine, but they may not supply these items. [Refer to Medicine, Ethics and Practice: a Guide for Pharmacists: midwives and controlled drugs.]

5 *Responding to symptoms:* Closed book

Section I

STYLE 1 – SIMPLE COMPLETION TYPE

5.1 **Answer D**

OTC hydrocortisone cream should not be sold for use in the following circumstances:

- broken or infected skin
- areas of the face, eye and anogenital region
- pregnancy (without medical advice)
- under 10 years of age (without medical advice)

5.2 **Answer E**

Widespread itching with yellowing of the skin may indicate jaundice, which requires the patient to be referred to their GP.

5.3 **Answer A**

Prophylaxis against malaria with chloroquine and proguanil should be used 1 week before entering the endemic area, for the whole duration of the stay, and for at least 4 weeks after leaving. [Refer to BNF 5.4.1 (antimalarials).]

5.4 **Answer C**

Symptoms of measles include:

- rash which is red-brown in colour and widespread, covering the neck, face and upper chest
- high temperature
- nasal discharge and conjunctivitis
- complaint of aching limbs
- white spots surrounded by a red ring present in the mouth

5.5 **Answer A**

OTC beclometasone nasal spray should be sold for the prevention and treatment of allergic rhinitis in adults aged over 18 years.

5.6 **Answer E**

Ringworm is a fungal infection that appears as circular skin lesions, with well-defined edges and central healing.

5.7 Answer D

Risk factors for coronary heart disease include: age, gender, family history, ethnicity, poverty, high intake of alcohol, high blood pressure, obesity, high serum cholesterol, high intake of fat, smoking and lack of physical exercise.

5.8 Answer C

Cow's milk has a higher content of protein and electrolytes, and lower amount of iron, compared to breast milk or infant feeds. Infants under 12 months of age should not be fed cow's milk.

5.9 Answer B

Rubella can cause fetal malformations during the early stages of pregnancy.

5.10 Answer E

Fungal infections involving the toenails require a prescription for oral antifungal treatment.

5.11 Answer C

Persistent coughs may be suggestive of serious illness, and referral to a medical practitioner may be required.

5.12 Answer E

Subconjunctival haemorrhages are self-limiting and not a serious condition.

5.13 Answer B

Cimetidine may be sold to adults (over 16 years) without prescription for short-term symptomatic relief of heartburn, dyspepsia, hyperacidity, and for prophylaxis of nocturnal heartburn.

5.14 Answer D

Omega-3 marine triglycerides present in oily fish can help to reduce plasma triglycerides.

5.15 Answer E

Candida albicans can cause thrush in the oral cavity. It is associated with the use of broad-spectrum antibacterials, cytotoxics, and ill-fitting dentures.

5.16 **Answer C**
Exacerbation of asthmatic symptoms requires referral to the GP.

5.17 **Answer B**
Chlorphenamine is an antihistamine.

5.18 **Answer D**
Symptoms of bacterial conjunctivitis include: redness of eyes; difficulty opening the eyes in the morning; and discharge from the eyes.

5.19 **Answer E**
Miconazole oral gel is indicated for the treatment of fungal infections of the lips, mouth and throat. It can be used for persons of any age.

5.20 **Answer E**
Miconazole cream 2% is used to treat fungal infections of the skin. It is applied twice a day and treatment continues for 10 days after the lesions have healed.

5.21 **Answer B**
Co-codaprin consists of aspirin and codeine. Paracetamol and paracetamol-containing preparations can be used with co-codaprin.

5.22 Answer B

The use of aspirin and NSAIDs in asthmatics is contraindicated as they may cause bronchoconstriction. Aspirin sensitivity occurs in approximately 10% of all asthmatic patients.

5.23 Answer A

Antimuscarinics are contraindicated in patients with angle-closure glaucoma, myasthenia gravis, paralytic ileus, pyloric stenosis and prostatic enlargement. [Refer to BNF 1.2 (antispasmodics and other drugs altering gut motility).]

5.24 Answer E *()*

The use of systemic decongestants is cautioned in the following conditions: diabetes, hypertension, hyperthyroidism, increased intraocular pressure, prostate hypertrophy, liver failure, renal failure and ischaemic heart disease. [Refer to BNF 3.10 (systemic nasal decongestants).]

5.25 Answer C

The incubation period of scabies is approximately 3 weeks. It is advisable that all members of the household be treated to prevent re-infestation from other household members.

5.26 Answer D

Shingles starts as small red lumps, producing a rash over the face and scalp.

5.27 Answer B

Impetigo is a contagious bacterial infection of the epidermis attributed to staphylococci or streptococci.

5.28 Answer B

Autoimmune gastritis leads to a deficiency in gastric intrinsic factor, which is required for the absorption of vitamin B_{12}. A lack of vitamin B_{12} causes pernicious anaemia.

5.29 Answer E

Vitamin E is present in vegetable oils.

5.30 Answer D
Vitamin D regulates the metabolism of calcium, including its absorption from the intestinal tract.

5.31 Answer C
Absorption of iron from plant sources is increased by taking vitamin C. Vegetarians should ensure that they have an intake of this vitamin.

5.32 Answer D
Vitamin D is obtained from dietary intake and is synthesised in the skin during exposure to sunlight.

5.33 Answer A
In order to reduce the risk of neural tube defects in the newborn, a folic acid dose, of 400 micrograms daily, should be taken by women before conception and during the first 12 weeks of pregnancy. [Refer to BNF 9.1.2 (drugs used in megaloblastic anaemias).]

5.34 Answer E
A hoarse voice lasting longer than 3 weeks may be suggestive of a serious condition, and referral to a GP is recommended in such situations.

5.35 Answer C
If a person has previously been diagnosed with haemorrhoids then a suitable preparation may be recommended. Referral to a GP is required if the symptoms have not improved within 7 days.

5.36 Answer E
Referral to a GP is required if cystitis presents with the following symptoms: loin pain; blood in the urine; fever; diabetes; nausea and vomiting; and recurrent symptoms.

5.37 Answer C
Where the cause of lower back pain has been identified (e.g. gardening, lifting) and the symptoms are not severe or debilitating, the patient should be advised to rest. If not contraindicated, an NSAID product may be used to reduce the pain and inflammation. Referral to a GP should be suggested if the symptoms have not improved within 1 week.

5.38 **Answer B**

Pseudoephedrine may reduce the effect of beta-blockers.

5.39 **Answer D**

Increased terfenadine concentrations are associated with rare hazardous arrhythmias.

5.40 **Answer C**

It can be difficult to assess whether sodium cromoglicate treatment will benefit a patient with asthma. The response should be evaluated after 4–6 weeks of treatment. [Refer to BNF 3.3.1 (cromoglicate and related therapy).]

5.41 **Answer D**

Initial treatment of diarrhoea in an infant is to prevent dehydration. Symptoms lasting longer than 1 day require the attention of a doctor.

5.42 **Answer E**

Diarrhoea following recent travel abroad may be infective in origin. Referral to a GP is required to determine the cause of the diarrhoea.

5.43 **Answer C**

Potassium is the main cation of intracellular fluid and is involved in carbohydrate metabolism, enzyme reactions, muscle contraction and nerve conduction.

5.44 **Answer A**

Calcium deficiency is likely to be brought about by a deficiency in vitamin D. Plasma calcium is regulated by vitamin D.

5.45 **Answer B**

Iron absorption from plant sources is improved by increasing the intake of vitamin C.

Section III

See Chapter 1 for key to responses for this section

5.46 Answer A

Antihistamine products licensed for the relief of temporary sleep disturbance should be used only when there is an identifiable cause to the disruption of normal sleep patterns, e.g. exam stress, long-haul flights and bereavement.

5.47 Answer A

Symptoms of meningitis include: headache, fever, nausea and vomiting, irritability, photophobia, confusion, skin rashes and neck stiffness.

5.48 Answer A

Folic acid intake should be greater than 400 micrograms per day in women who are planning to become pregnant and who are associated with one of the following:

- a child with spina bifida by either partner

- a history of neural tube defect in a previous child

- the woman is receiving regular anti-epileptic therapy

[Refer to BNF 9.1.2 (drugs used in megaloblastic anaemia).]

5.49 Answer D

Drugs which exhibit antimuscarinic actions may cause side-effects of constipation, dry mouth, drowsiness, dizziness, blurred vision and difficulty passing urine.

5.50 **Answer A**

Self-treatment of thrush is not advisable, but referral to a GP, for the following women:

- first-time sufferers of thrush
- those in whom two attacks of thrush have occurred in the previous 6 months
- those who are pregnant or breast-feeding
- those aged under 16 years or over 60 years
- those with blood-stained vaginal discharge
- those with abdominal pain
- those with pain or difficulty in passing urine
- those who have seen no improvement of symptoms within 7 days of using an appropriate OTC product

5.51 **Answer C**

Diabetics with foot problems and men with cystitis need to be referred to a doctor for assessment.

5.52 **Answer A**

Threadworm infestations, in people over 2 years of age, should be treated with mebendazole. Further measures to help reduce the presence of threadworm eggs include: practising good hygiene measures (e.g. washing hands before eating and after going to the toilet; washing bed linen and towels frequently), frequent vacuuming of the home; and an early morning shower or bath. [Refer to BNF 5.5.1 (drugs for threadworm).]

5.53 **Answer B**

Constipation is a possible side-effect of drugs that have an antimuscarinic action. Antimuscarinics reduce intestinal bowel movement. [Refer to BNF 1.2 (antispasmodics and other drugs altering gut motility).]

5.54 **Answer B**

Drugs which can reduce the effect of oral contraceptives include those which induce hepatic enzyme activity and certain antibacterials. Additional contraceptive precautions should be advised in patients taking such drugs. [Refer to BNF 7.3.1 (combined hormonal contraceptives).]

5.55 **Answer A**

A migraine attack may be treated with simple analgesics (aspirin, paracetamol, NSAIDs), with possible addition of an anti-emetic (domperidone, metoclopramide). Further treatment may involve the use of $5HT_1$ agonists (naratriptan, sumatriptan, zolmitriptan). Ergot alkaloids (ergotamine) are rarely used in the treatment of migraines. [Refer to BNF 4.7.4.1 (treatment of the acute migraine attack).]

5.56 **Answer C**

Symptoms of chest pain and shortness of breath are suggestive of a more serious condition; thus, the patient requires a referral to a GP.

5.57 **Answer E**

Some people may be asymptomatic during the early stages of threadworm infection. All members of the household should be treated at the same time to prevent re-infection. [Refer to BNF 5.5.1 (drugs for threadworms).]

5.58 **Answer D**

Blood in vomit is indicative of a serious condition and referral to a GP is required.

5.59 **Answer A**

Smoking is a risk factor associated with several conditions, including heart disease, peptic ulcers and bronchitis.

5.60 **Answer C**

The characteristics of classical migraine include:

- three times more common in women than in men
- visual disturbances often occur in the prodromal phase
- some relief from an attack may be obtained by lying in a darkened room

5.61 **Answer B**

OTC hydrocortisone cream should not be sold for use in the following circumstances:

- broken or infected skin
- areas of the face, eye and anogenital region
- pregnancy (without medical advice)
- under 10 years of age (without medical advice)

5.62 **Answer A**

Pregnant women should:

- avoid eating soft unpasteurised cheese as it may harbour *Listeria*, which can harm the fetus or cause a miscarriage
- avoid eating sources that have a high vitamin A content (e.g. liver), which is teratogenic
- avoid contact with cat litter because of the risk of contracting toxoplasmosis, which can harm the fetus

5.63 **Answer D**

Aspirin is contraindicated in children and adolescents under the age of 16 years, due to the risk of Reye's syndrome (unless specifically indicated).

5.64 **Answer C**

First aid treatment of minor burns is as follows:

- remove jewellery or any articles which may restrict blood flow
- cool the affected area with running water for 15 minutes
- do not apply any creams or ointments
- blisters should not be burst due to the risk of infection and scarring
- cover with clingfilm or a clean, dry, non-fluffy cotton cloth
- take simple analgesics for pain relief

5.65 **Answer A**

All members of the family should be checked for head lice and treated at the same time. Alcohol-based products should be avoided in asthmatics (risk of wheezing) and in people with severe eczema (risk of skin inflammation).

Section IV

See Chapter 1 for key to responses for this section

5.66 Answer C
The emergency hormonal contraceptive (EHC) may be used more than once within one menstrual cycle. Providing advice about methods of contraception is part of good practice when counselling on EHC. [Refer to BNF 7.3.1 (combined hormonal contraceptives).]

5.67 Answer D
Lotions or liquid preparations should be used to treat head lice; the dilution of shampoos while in use lessens their effect. Aqueous preparations are preferred in small children, asthmatics, and in patients who have severe eczema. BNF 13.10.4 (parasiticidal preparations).]

5.68 Answer D
Five portions of fruit and vegetables are required for a healthy diet. Antioxidants are present in fruit and vegetables, which may help to prevent or delay the occurrence of cancer and atherosclerosis.

5.69 Answer E
Pregnant women are not advised to take vitamin A supplements (e.g. cod-liver oil) or foods with a high content of vitamin A (e.g. liver) due to the risk of teratogeneticity. [Refer to BNF 9.6.1 (vitamin A).]

5.70 Answer C
Folic acid supplements should be taken by women planning to become pregnant and during the first trimester of pregnancy. Smoking does not reduce folic acid levels. [Refer to BNF 9.1.2 (drugs used in megaloblastic anaemias).]

5.71 Answer E
Nicotine gum is to be chewed for 30 minutes to release all available nicotine.

5.72 **Answer D**

Pregnant women are not advised to take vitamin A supplements (e.g. cod-liver oil) or foods with a high content of vitamin A (e.g. liver), due to risk of teratogeneticity. [Refer to BNF 9.6.1 (vitamin A).]

5.73 **Answer B**

Warts (verrucas) are caused by a human papillomavirus. Treatment using OTC preparations include salicyclic acid, formaldehyde, glutaraldehyde and silver nitrate. [Refer to BNF 13.7 (preparations for warts and calluses).]

5.74 **Answer A**

Foods rich in vitamin B_{12} are liver, meat, fish and eggs. Yeast extracts are a suitable alternative for strict vegetarians.

5.75 **Answer D**

Replacing and preventing fluid and electrolyte loss is the priority for diarrhoea. Oral rehydration preparations fulfil this requirement and are suitable for diabetes. [Refer to BNF 1.4 (acute diarrhoea).]

5 *Responding to Symptoms:* Open book

STYLE 1 – SIMPLE COMPLETION TYPE

5.76 **Answer E**
H_2-antagonists may be sold to the public (except ranitidine bismuth citrate) provided packs do not contain more than 14 days' supply.

5.77 **Answer E**
Cough suppressants are cautioned in patients with asthma.

5.78 **Answer A**
Sedating antihistamines are cautioned in patients with urinary retention, glaucoma, prostatic hypertrophy, pyloroduodenal obstruction, liver disease, kidney failure (reduce dose) and epilepsy. Children and the elderly may be susceptible to the side-effects of antihistamines. [Refer to BNF 3.4.1 (antihistamines).]

5.79 **Answer C**
[Refer to BNF 5.4.1 (antimalarials).]

5.80 **Answer C**
Decongestant nasal products for the relief of nasal congestion should not be used for longer than 7 days; there is a risk of rebound congestion if used for longer periods. [Refer to BNF 12.2.2 (topical nasal decongestants).]

5.81 **Answer B**
Derbac-M® is a suitable product to sell without prescription for treating head lice in asthmatics. Alcohol-based products should be avoided in asthmatics due to the risk of wheezing.

5.82 **Answer A**
Alginates form a 'raft' on top of stomach contents and are useful in protecting against gastro-oesophageal reflux disease. Low-sodium products are recommended for patients on a low-salt diet or with heart disease or hypertension to ensure that the acid balance of the blood is not upset. [Refer to BNF 1.1 (dyspepsia and gastro-oesophageal reflux disease).]

5.83 Answer C

Difflam® (benzydamine) oral rinse is indicated for the relief of painful inflammatory conditions of the mouth and throat. [Refer to BNF 12.3.4 (mouthwashes, gargles, and dentifrices).]

5.84 Answer E

Aspirin and NSAIDs should be avoided in patients with dyspepsia, and gastric and duodenal ulcers (unless specifically indicated). [Refer to BNF 1.3 (ulcer-healing drugs).]

5.85 Answer E

Prevention and reversal of fluid and electrolyte loss is the priority in acute diarrhoea. Oral rehydration preparations are first-line treatments in acute diarrhoea. [Refer to BNF 1.4 (acute diarrhoea).]

STYLE 2 – CLASSIFICATION TYPE

5.86 Answer B
Promethazine is the most sedating antihistamine available
without prescription for preventing motion sickness. OTC
preparations containing promethazine include Avomine®,
Phenergan® and Phenergan Elixir®. [Refer to BNF 4.6 (drugs
used in nausea and vertigo).]

5.87 Answer A
Hyoscine is the effective drug for the prevention of motion
sickness. OTC preparations containing hyoscine include Joy-
Rides®, Kwells® and Kwells Junior®. [Refer to BNF 4.6 (drugs
used in nausea and vertigo).]

5.88 Answer B
Buclizine is an ingredient in Migraleve Pink® (an OTC
product for the treatment of migraine attacks).

5.89 Answer E
Promethazine is available in OTC preparations for the short-
term correction of insomnia. [Refer to BNF 4.1.1 (hypnotics).]

5.90 Answer A
Cyproheptadine is an antihistamine that has an indication for
migraine. [Refer to BNF 4.7.4.2 (prophylaxis of migraine).]

5.91 Answer B
Simeticone is added to some antacid preparations and acts as
an antifoaming agent to relieve flatulence. [Refer to BNF 1.1.1
(antacids and simeticone).]

5.92 Answer E
Antacids consisting of magnesium salts also relieve
constipation due to their laxative effect. [Refer to BNF 1.1.1
(antacids and simeticone).]

5.93 Answer C
Alginates are added to some antacids and act by forming a
'raft' on top of stomach contents and are useful in protecting
against gastro-oesophageal reflux disease. [Refer to BNF 1.1.1
(antacids and simeticone).]

5.94 **Answer E**

Terbinafine 1% cream may be sold without prescription for the external treatment of athlete's foot (tinea pedis) and dhobie itch (tinea cruris). [Refer to BNF 13.10.2 (antifungal preparations).]

5.95 **Answer A**

Dimeticone is a water-repellant and is added to some barrier preparations. [Refer to BNF 13.2.2 (barrier preparations).]

5.96 **Answer B**

Hydrocortisone butyrate is generally required in patients with severe eczemas, which tend to be unresponsive to less potent topical corticosteroids. [Refer to BNF 13.4 (topical corticosteroids).]

STYLE 3 – MULTIPLE COMPLETION TYPE

See Chapter 1 for key to responses for this section

5.97 **Answer D**

There is an increased risk of hyperkalaemia when potassium salts are taken with ACE inhibitors. Preparations containing pseudoephedrine are not recommended to be used in patients with hypertension.

5.98 **Answer D**

Folic acid, in amounts greater than 400 micrograms, should be taken by women who are receiving anti-epileptic medication and who are planning to become, or are, pregnant. [Refer to BNF 9.1.2 (drugs used in megaloblastic anaemias).]

5.99 **Answer E**

The use of systemic decongestants is cautioned in the following conditions: diabetes, hypertension, hyperthyroidism, increased intra-ocular pressure, prostate hypertrophy, liver failure, renal failure, and ischaemic heart disease. [Refer to BNF 3.10 (systemic nasal decongestants).]

5.100 **Answer E**

The use of aspirin and NSAIDs should be avoided during pregnancy, unless indicated by the direction of a medical practitioner. [Refer to BNF Appendix 4 (pregnancy).]

5.101 **Answer C**

Piperazine is to be avoided in patients with epilepsy. [Refer to BNF 5.5.1 (drugs for threadworms).]

5.102 **Answer B**

Betoptic® (betaxolol) is a topical beta-blocker used to reduce intra-ocular pressure in glaucoma. Drugs which have an antimuscarinic action should not be used in patients with glaucoma.

5.103 **Answer A**

The use of systemic decongestants is cautioned in the following conditions: diabetes, hypertension, hyperthyroidism, increased intra-ocular pressure, prostate hypertrophy, liver failure, renal failure, and ischaemic heart disease. [Refer to BNF 3.10 (systemic nasal decongestants).]

See Chapter 1 for key to responses for this section

5.104 **Answer A**

Pholcodine is indicated for dry or painful cough and may be used by diabetics. [Refer to BNF 3.9.1 (cough suppressants).]

5.105 **Answer A**

Amitriptyline and chlorpheniramine both have antimuscarinic side-effects. There is an increased risk of antimuscarinic and sedative effects when antihistamines and tricyclic antidepressants are given together. [Refer to BNF Appendix 1 (interactions).]

5.106 **Answer A**

The incidence of antimuscarinic side-effects is lower in non-sedating antihistamines than in sedating antihistamines. [Refer to BNF 3.4.1 (antihistamines).]

5.107 **Answer A**

Potassium citrate causes alkalisation of urine and should not be used in patients taking methenamine. Methenamine requires acidic urine for its action against bacteria. [Refer to BNF Appendix 1 (interactions).]

6 Calculations

Section I

STYLE 1 – SIMPLE COMPLETION TYPE

6.1 **Answer C**

400 ml equal parts rose water and witch hazel
= (200 ml rose water) + (200 ml witch hazel)
Concentrate is 40 times single strength
200 ml ÷ 40 = 5 ml of concentrated rose water required

6.2 **Answer C**

Total weight = (400 g of water) + (44.4 g of solid)
= 444.4 g
10% w/w = 444.4 g × (10 ÷ 100)
= 44.4 g of sodium carbonate

6.3 **Answer B**

0.25% w/w = 250 mg in 100 g
Therefore in 600 g
250 mg × 6 = 1500 mg or 1.5 g of aqueous cream 0.25% w/w required

6.4 **Answer D**

(0.8 ÷ 2.5) × 100 g = 32 g of hydrocortisone cream 2.5% required

6.5 **Answer C**

0.5% w/v ≡ 1 in 200 solution
Dilution factor = 40
Volume = 2000 ml ÷ 40
= 50 ml of 0.5% w/v stock solution is required

6.6 **Answer B**

Fersamal® syrup is 45 mg ferrous iron in 5 ml
Dose = 2.4 ml × 2.0 kg = 4.8 ml
Amount of ferrous iron = (4.8 ÷ 5) × 45 mg
= 43.2 mg of ferrous iron daily

6.7 **Answer A** ↑

Dose of Fucidin® suspension for a child up to 1 year is 50 mg/kg daily (in 3 divided doses)
Daily dose required = 50 mg × 5.4 kg = 270 mg
Max. single dose = 270 mg ÷ 3 = 90 mg
Fucidin® suspension is 250 mg per 5 ml
Volume of single dose = (90 ÷ 250) × 5 ml
= 1.8 ml of Fucidin® suspension

6.8 **Answer C**

1 litre of glucose 5% infusion contains 50 g glucose in 1000 ml
1 litre of KCl, NaCl and glucose intravenous infusion contains 40 g glucose in 1000 ml (i.e. 4% glucose)
Total amount of glucose = 50 g + 40 g
= 90 g glucose given over 24 hours

6.9 **Answer B**

Total weight = (1 g sodium bicarbonate) + (10 g water) = 11 g
Strength of solution = (1 ÷ 11) = 9.09 %w/w

6.10 **Answer E**

12.5 w/w = 12.5 g in 100 g
Therefore in 280 g
(12.5 ÷ 100) × 280 g = 35 g of emulsifying wax

6.11 **Answer C**

Lower limit = (90 ÷ 100) × 200 mg = 180 mg
Upper limit = (110 ÷ 100) × 200 mg = 220 mg
Range = 180 – 220 mg

6.12 **Answer D** ↑

Dose of proguanil required: 200 mg once daily, starting 1 week before travel into an endemic area, and continued for at least 4 weeks after leaving. [Refer to BNF 5.4.1 (antimalarials).]
Total number of proguanil tablets 100 mg to supply
= 7 weeks or 49 days total supply required
= 49 × 2 = 98 proguanil tablets 100 mg required

6.13 **Answer E**

One Bricanyl® tablet contains 5 mg terbutaline sulphate
Bricanyl® syrup is 1.5 mg terbutaline sulphate per 5 ml.
Amount of Bricanyl® syrup equivalent to one Bricanyl® tablet is:

$(5 \div 1.5) \times 5$ ml = 16.67 ml of Bricanyl® syrup

6.14 **Answer E**

1 in 200 ≡ 1 g in 200 ml
Amount required in 1 litre:
$(1000 \div 200) \times 1$ g = 5 g of potassium permanganate

6.15 **Answer E**

Chlorphenamine syrup is 2 mg in 5 ml
Daily volume required = $(5 \div 2)$ mg × 5 ml × 3 doses= 37.5 ml
Total volume to supply = 37.5 ml × 8 days = 300 ml

6.16 Answer D
Loratadine syrup is 5 mg/5 ml.
40 ml of loratadine syrup contains 40 mg loratadine

6.17 Answer B
0.4% KCl solution consists of 0.4 g of potassium chloride in
100 ml

6.18 Answer B
1 in 1000 = 1 g in 1000 ml
Therefore,
(200 ÷ 1000) × 1 g = 0.2 g of potassium citrate powder required

6.19 Answer C
0.05 % = 0.05 g in 100 ml
Therefore,
(4000 ÷ 100) × 0.05 g = 2 g of potassium citrate powder
required

6.20 Answer D
Max. dose of ibuprofen in juvenile rheumatoid arthritis in chil-
dren over 7 kg: 40 mg/kg daily in 3 or 4 divided doses
Ideal body weight for a 1 year old = 10 kg
Daily dose = 40 mg × 10 kg = 400 mg
Possible divided doses:
400 mg ÷ 3 = 133 mg t.d.s.
400 mg ÷ 4 = 100 mg q.d.s.
Only available choice from answer options is 100 mg q.d.s.

6.21 Answer C
Clindamycin dose in severe infections in a child over 1 month
is 300 mg daily (regardless of weight), which is equivalent to
100 mg t.d.s.

6.22 Answer C B

Usual intramuscular dose of cefuroxime in children is
60 mg/kg daily in 3 or 4 divided doses
Daily dose = 60 mg × 3 kg = 180mg
Possible divided doses:
180 mg ÷ 3 = 60 mg t.d.s.
180 mg ÷ 4 = 45 mg q.d.s.
Only available choice from answer options is 60 mg t.d.s.

6.23 Answer C

Aromatic magnesium carbonate mixture BP contains sodium
bicarbonate 5%
Therefore, amount of sodium bicarbonate 5% in 600 ml aromatic magnesium carbonate BP is:
(600 ÷ 100) × 5 g = 30 g of sodium bicarbonate 5%

6.24 Answer B

Kaolin and morphine mixture BP contains sodium bicarbonate
5%
Therefore, amount of sodium bicarbonate 5% in 60 ml kaolin
and morphine mixture BP is:
(60 ÷ 100) × 5 g = 3 g of sodium bicarbonate 5%

6.25 Answer A

Low Na^+ indicates a sodium content of less than 1 mmol per
tablet or 10 ml dose. [Refer to BNF 1.1.1 (antacids and simeticone).]

6.26 Answer E

Physiological saline is sodium chloride 0.9% (9 g, 150 mmol
each of Na^+ and Cl^- per litre)
Number of mmol of sodium equivalent to 60 g of sodium chloride is:
(60 ÷ 9) × 150 mmol = 1000 mmol of sodium

Section III

See Chapter 1 for key to responses for this section

6.27 Answer C

100 microgram/ml solution = 0.1 mg in 1 ml
∴ 0.3 mg in 3 ml
1 in 1000 solution = 1 mg in 1 ml
∴ 0.3 mg in 0.3 ml
1 in 10 000 solution = 1 mg in 10 ml
∴ 0.3 mg in 3 ml

6.28 Answer D

Subcutaneous dose of pentazocaine, for a child over 1 year, is given up to 1 mg/kg
Ideal body weight of a 5-year-old child is 18 kg
Each dose required = 1 mg × 18 kg = 18 mg
Hence, any amount up to 18 mg may be given.
0.5 ml of 30 mg/ml injection = 15 mg
0.7 ml of 30 mg/ml injection = 21 mg
1.0 ml of 30 mg/ml injection = 30 mg

6.29 Answer A

Single dose of intramuscular pethidine in a child is 0.5–2.0 mg/kg
Ideal body weight of a 3-year-old is 15 kg
Dose range is 7.5–30 mg; doses within this range are suitable for administration
0.8 ml of 10 mg/ml injection = 8 mg
0.3 ml of 50 mg/ml injection = 15 mg
0.6 ml of 50 mg/ml injection = 30 mg

6.30 Answer D

Each Calcichew® contains calcium 500 mg
∴ 1 tablet o.d. ≡ 500 mg daily
5 ml Calcium-Sandoz® syrup contains calcium 108.3 mg
∴ 5 ml t.d.s. ≡ 324.9 mg daily
Each Ossopan® tablet contains calcium 178 mg
∴ 1 tablet o.d. ≡ 178 mg daily

6.31 Answer D

2 Fersaday® tablets ≡ 200 mg iron
2 Feospan® capsules ≡ 94 mg iron
2 Fersamal® tablets ≡ 136 mg iron

STYLE 4 –ASSERTION–REASON TYPE

See Chapter 1 for key to responses for this section

6.32 **Answer A**

Initial infusion rate of lidocaine is 4 mg/minute or 240 mg/ hour

Lidocaine 0.2% solution ≡ 0.2 g in 100 ml

∴ 240 mg in 120 ml

∴ Infusion rate is set at 120 ml/hour

6.33 **Answer A**

Sodium bicarbonate 8.4 %w/v solution ≡ 8.4 g in 100 ml

Therefore, in 3 litre (3000 ml):

(3000 ÷ 100) × 8.4 g = 252 g of sodium bicarbonate

12.6 g of sodium bicarbonate contains 150 mmol of both sodium and bicarbonate ions

∴ 3 litres ≡ (252 ÷ 12.6) × 150 mmol

≡ 3000 mmol of ions in 3000 ml

≡ 1 mmol in 1 ml

6.34 **Answer D**

25 mg in 12.5 ml

∴ 200 mg in 100 ml ≡ 8% w/v

i.e. 2 mg in 1 ml

8 Appendices

Appendix I: Abbreviations of health and pharmacy organisations and technical terms

Abbreviation	Term
ABPI	Association of the British Pharmaceutical Industry
ACBS	Advisory Committee on Borderline Substances
ATO	Assistant technical officer
BAN	British Approved Name
BMA	British Medical Association
BNF	British National Formulary (latest edition should be used, unless otherwise stated)
BP	British Pharmacopoeia (latest edition should be used, unless otherwise stated)
BPC	British Pharmaceutical Codex 1973 and Supplement 1976, unless otherwise stated
BPSA	British Pharmaceutical Students' Association
CCA	Company Chemists Association
CD	Controlled drug (designated preparations are controlled by the Misuse of Drugs Act 1971 and are subject to the prescription requirements under the Misuse of Drugs Regulations 2001)
CD Anab	Controlled drug: anabolic and androgenic steroids (Schedule 4 Part II drugs)
CD Benz	Controlled drug: benzodiazepines (Schedule 4 Part I drugs)
CD Inv.	Controlled drug: invoice (Schedule 5 drugs)
CD Lic	Controlled drug: licence (Schedule 1 drugs) – the production, possession and supply of such drugs requires a Home Office licence
CD No Reg	Controlled drug: no register (Schedule 3 drugs)
CDSM	Committee on Dental and Surgical Materials
CHI	Commission for Health Improvement (ceased operating on 31 March 2004; functions taken over by the Healthcare Commission)
CHIP	Chemicals Hazard Information and Packaging for supply [certain chemicals must comply with the Chemical (Hazard Information and Packaging Supply) Regulations 2002]
CP	Calendar pack
CPA	Commonwealth Pharmaceutical Association
CPD	Continuing Professional Development
CPMP	Committee on Proprietary Medicinal Products

CPP	College of Pharmacy Practice
CPPE	Centre for Pharmacy Postgraduate Education
CRM	Committee on the Review of Medicines
CSM	Committee on Safety of Medicines
DEB	denatured ethanol B
DEFRA	Department for Environment, Food and Rural Affairs
DoH	Department of Health
DPF	Dental Practitioners' Formulary
EMEA	European Medicines Evaluation Agency
GDC	General Dental Council
GLP	Good laboratory practice
GMC	General Medical Council
GMP	Good Manufacturing Practice
GP	General Practitioner
GSL	General Sale List medicine
HO	House officer (hospital doctor)
IMS	industrial methylated spirits
INN	International non-proprietary name
JHO	Junior house officer (grade of hospital doctor)
MA	Marketing Authorisation
MCA	Medicines Control Agency (now MHRA)
MEP	Medicines, Ethics and Practice: a Guide for Pharmacists (latest edition should be used, unless otherwise stated)
MFS	Medicated feedingstuffs prescription
MFSX	Exemption from medicated feedstuffs prescription
MHRA	Medicines and Healthcare products Regulatory Agency
MI	Medicines information
MMS	mineralised methylated spirits
NatPaCT	National Primary and Care Trust Development Programme
NCL	no cautionary labels
NHS	National Health Service
NICE	National Institute for Clinical Excellence
NMC	Nurse and Midwifery Council
NP	proper name
NPA	National Pharmaceutical Association
NPC	National Prescribing Centre
NPF	Nurse Prescribers' Formulary
NPSA	National Patient Safety Agency
NSF	National Service Framework
OTC	over-the-counter medicine
P	Pharmacy medicine(s)
PA	Patients' Association

PACT	Prescribing Analysis and CosT
PGD	patient group direction
PHLS	Public Health Laboratory Service
PIL	patient information leaflet
PL	Product Licence (now MA)
PML	Pharmacy and merchant list
PMR	patient medication record
PO	Pharmacy-only medicine
POM	Prescription-only medicines
PPA	Prescription Pricing Authority
PSNC	Pharmaceutical Services Negotiating Committee
PSRP	Patient Safety Research Programme
QA	Quality Assurance
rINN	Recommended International Non-proprietary Name
RN	Registered nurse
RPSGB	Royal Pharmaceutical Society of Great Britain
SHO	Senior house officer (grade of hospital doctor)
SIGN	Scottish Intercollegiate Guidelines Network
SLS	Selected List Scheme
SMAC	Standing Medical Advisory Committee
SOPs	standard operating procedures
SPC	Summary of Product Characteristics
UK	United Kingdom
UKCPA	UK Clinical Pharmacy Association
UKMi	UK Medicines Information
USP	United States Pharmacopeia (latest edition should be used, unless otherwise stated)
WADA	World Anti-Doping Agency
WHO	World Health Organisation
WWHAM	Mnemonic used for over-the-counter sales of medicines: Who is the medicine for? What is the medicine for? How long have the symptoms been present? Action already taken? Medicines taken for other reason, prescribed or otherwise?
YPG	Young Pharmacists Group

Appendix II: **Symbols used in pharmacy**

▼	'Black triangle' symbol – identifies newly licensed medicines and/or products with limited experience of use; MHRA/CSM intensively monitors these items and requests that all suspected adverse reactions be reported
◩	Identifies products considered by the Joint Formulary Committee to be less suitable for prescribing
®	Registered trade mark
Δ	Diagnosis
ΔΔ	Differential diagnosis
°	Absent
†	Died
#	Fracture
∴	Therefore
∵	Because
-ve, −	Negative
+ve, +	Positive
↔	No change
1°	Primary
2°	Secondary
1/7	One day
1/52	One week
1/12	One month

Appendix III: Latin terms and abbreviations

Prescription directions should be written in English, without the use of abbreviations. However, some prescribers use Latin terms and abbreviations to indicate the dosage form and frequency of the preparation. The following is a list of common terms and abbreviations that may be encountered in pharmacy practice. The English term is not always a literal translation of the Latin word.

Latin	Abbreviation	Term
ad	ad	to
ad libitum	ad lib.	as much as desired
alternus	alt.	alternate
ana	a.a.	of each
ante	ante	before
ante cibum	a.c.	before food
ante meridiem	a.m.	before noon
applicandus	applic.	to be applied
aqua	aq.	water
auristillae	aurist.	ear drops
bis	b.	twice
bis die	b.d.	twice daily
bis in die	b.i.d.	twice daily
capsula	caps.	capsule
cataplasma	cataplasm.	poultice
cibus	cib.	food
collutorium	collut.	mouthwash
collyrium	collyr.	eye lotion
compositus	co.	compound
concentratus	conc.	concentrated
cremor	crem.	cream
cum	c.	with
destillatus	dest.	distilled
dies	d.	a day
dilutus	dil.	diluted
duplex	dup.	double
ex aqua	ex aq.	in water
fiat	ft.	let it be made
fortis	fort.	strong
guttae	gtt.	drops
haustus	ht.	draught

hora	h.	at the hour of
hora somni	h.s.	at bedtime
inter	int.	between
inter cibos	i.c.	between meals
liquor	liq.	solution
lotio	lot.	lotion
mane	m.	in the morning
mistura	mist.	mixture
mitte	mitt.	send
more dicto	m.d.	as directed
more dicto utendus	m.d.u.	to be used as directed
naristillae	narist.	nose drops
nebula	neb.	nebuliser (spray) solution
nocte	n./noct.	at night
nocte et mane	n. et m.	night and morning
nocte maneque	n.m.	night and morning
nomen proprium	n.p.	proper name
oculentum	oculent.	eye ointment
omni die	o.d.	daily
omni mane	o.m.	every morning
omni nocte	o.n	every night
omnibus alternis horis	o.alt.hor	every other hour
partes	pp.	parts
partes aequales	p. aeq.	equal parts
parti affectae	p.a.	to the affected part
parti affectae applicandus	part. affect.	to be applied to the affected part
pasta	past.	paste
pigmentum	pig.	paint
post cibum	p.c.	after food
post meridiem	p.m.	afternoon
pro re nata	p.r.n.	when required
pulvis	pulv.	powder
pulvis conspersus	pulv. consp.	dusting powder
quantum sufficiat	q.s.	sufficient
quaque	qq.	every
quaque hora	qq.h.	every hour
quarta quaque hora	q.q.h.	every 4 hours
quater die	q.d.	four times daily
quater die sumendus	q.d.s.	to be taken four times daily
quater in die	q.i.d.	four times daily
recipe	Rx	take
semisse	ss.	half

si opus sit	s.o.s.	if necessary
signa	sig.	label
statim	stat.	immediately
sumendus ter	sum. t.	to be taken three times
ter de die	t.d.d.	three time daily
ter die sumendus	t.d.s.	to be taken three times daily
ter in die	t.i.d.	three times daily
trochiscus	troch.	lozenge
tussi urgente	tuss. urg.	when the cough troubles
tussis	tuss.	cough
unguentum	ung.	ointment
urgente	urg.	urgent
ut antea	u.a.	as before
ut dictum	ut. dict.	as directed
ut directum	ut. direct.	as directed
utendus	utend.	to be used
vapor	vap.	inhalation

Appendix IV: Abbreviations used in medical notes

Abbreviation	Term
ACE	angiotensin-converting enzyme
ADHD	attention deficit hyperactivity disorder
ADR	adverse drug reaction
AF	atrial fibrillation
AIDS	acquired immunodeficiency syndrome
ALL	acute lymphocytic leukaemia
ALT	alanine aminotransferase
AML	acute myeloid leukaemia
AP	anteroposterior
approx.	approximately
appt.	appointment
ARF	acute renal failure
AV	atrioventricular
AXR	abdominal X-ray
BCG	bacillus Calmette–Guérin (vaccine)
BMI	body mass index
BP	blood pressure
BPH	benign prostatic hypertrophy
bpm	beats per minute
BSA	body surface area
c	with (Latin: *cum*)
C/I	contraindications
c/o	complains of
c/r	controlled-release
CA, Ca, ca	cancer
CABG	coronary artery bypass graft
CAD	coronary artery disease
CAPD	continuous ambulatory peritoneal dialysis
caps.	capsules
CCF	congestive cardiac failure
CCU	Coronary Care Unit
CF	cystic fibrosis
CHD	congenital heart disease
CHF	congestive heart failure
CK	creatinine kinase
CLL	chronic lymphocytic leukaemia
CMV	cytomegalovirus
CNS	central nervous system

COAD	chronic obstructive airway disease
COPD	chronic obstructive pulmonary disease
CPK	creatinine phosphokinase
CRF	chronic renal failure
CRP	C-reactive protein
CSF	cerebrospinal fluid
CT	computerised tomography
CVS	cardiovascular system
CXR	chest X-ray
D&V	diarrhoea and vomiting
D/I	drug interactions
DH	drug history
DM	diabetes mellitus
DNA	did not attend
DNR	do not resuscitate
DOB	date of birth
DOE	dyspnoea on exertion
DPT	diphtheria, pertussis, tetanus (vaccine)
DVT	deep vein thrombosis
Dx	diagnosis
e/c	enteric-coated (also known as gastro-resistant)
ECF	extracellular fluid
ECG	electrocardiogram
ECT	electroconvulsive therapy
EHC	emergency hormonal contraception
ENT	ear, nose and throat
ESR	erythrocyte sedimentation rate
f/c	film-coated
FBC	full blood count
FFA	free fatty acids
FH	family history
FU	follow-up
FUO	fever of unknown origin
FVC	force vital capacity
Fx	fracture
G6PD	glucose 6-phosphate dehydrogenase
GA	general anaesthetic
GCS	Glasgow Coma Scale
GFR	glomerular filtration rate
GI(T)	gastrointestinal (tract)
GORD	gastro-oesophageal reflux disease
GTN	glyceryl trinitrate
GTT	glucose tolerance test

GU	genitourinary
GYN	gynaecology
Hb	haemoglobin
HCG	human chorionic gonadotrophin
HDL	high-density lipoprotein
HDU	High Dependency Unit
Hep	hepatitis
HIV	human immunodeficiency virus
HL	Hodgkin's lymphoma
HLA	human leukocyte antigen
HPI	history of presenting illness
HR	heart rate
HRT	hormone replacement therapy
Hx	history
i/m, i.m.	intramuscular
i/v, i.v.	intravenous
IBS	irritable bowel syndrome
ICF	intracellular fluid
ICU	Intensive Care Unit
IHD	ischaemic heart disease
inj	injection
INR	international normalised ratio (prothrombin time)
INT	drug interactions
IP	inpatient
ITU	intensive therapy unit
IUD	intrauterine device
Ix	investigations
JVP	jugular venous pulse
KUB	kidneys, ureters, bladder
LA	local anaesthetic
LDH	lactate dehydrogenase
LDL	low-density lipoprotein
LFTs	liver function tests
LVF	left ventricular failure
LVH	left ventricular hypertrophy
LWBS	left without being seen
m.d.	maximum dose
m.d.d.	maximum daily dose
m.s.	maximum strength
m/r	modified-release
MAOIs	monoamine oxidase inhibitors
MAP	mean arterial pressure
max.	maximum

MCH	mean corpuscular haemoglobin
MCHC	mean corpuscular haemoglobin concentration
MCV	mean corpuscular volume
MI	myocardial infarction
min.	minimum
MMR	mumps, measles, rubella (vaccine)
MRI	magnetic resonance imaging
MRSA	methicillin-resistant *Staphylococcus aureus*
MS	multiple sclerosis
N&V	nausea and vomiting
NBM	Nil by mouth
neb.	nebuliser solution (Latin: *nebula*)
NHL	non-Hodgkin's lymphoma
NICU	neonatal intensive care unit
NKA	no known allergies
NSAID	non-steroidal anti-inflammatory drug
O/A	on admission
O/E	on examination
OP	outpatient
OT	occupational therapy
p.o.	per oral
p.r.	per rectum
p.v.	per vagina
PA	posteroanterior
PC	presenting complaint
PCV	packed cell volume
PD	Parkinson's disease
PD	peritoneal dialysis
PE	pulmonary embolus
PEF(R)	peak expiratory flow (rate)
PET	positron emission tomography
PFR	peak flow rate
PG	prostaglandin
PH	past history
PKU	phenylketonuria
PMH	past medical history
PMS	premenstrual syndrome
PN	parenteral nutrition
PT	prothrombin time
PTA	prior to admission
PTCA	percutaneous transluminal coronary angioplasty
PVD	peripheral vascular disease
r/c	rubber capped (vial)

RBC	red blood cell/count
RF	renal failure
RHD	rheumatic heart disease
RICE	Rest, Ice, Compression and Elevation (first aid mnemonic for musculoskeletal injuries)
RSV	respiratory syncytial virus
RV	residual volume
Rx	recipe (Latin: *take*; commonly denotes prescription)
S&S	signs and symptoms
s.c.	subcutaneous
S/B	seen by
s/c	sugar-coated
S/P	special precautions
SA	sino-atrial
SBO	small bowel obstruction
SCBU	Special Care Baby Unit
SH	social history
SLE	systemic lupus erythematosus
SOB	shortness of breath
spp.	species
SSRIs	selective serotonin re-uptake inhibitors
stat	immediately (Latin: *statim*)
STD	sexually transmitted disease
sust. release	sustained-release
Sx	symptoms
SXR	skull X-ray
T_3	tri-iodothyronine
T_4	(levo)thyroxine
tabs.	tablets
TB	tuberculosis
TFTs	thyroid function tests
TIA	transient ischaemic attack
TLC	total lung capacity
TPN	total parenteral nutrition
TPR	temperature, pulse, respirations
TTAs	to take away (discharge medicines)
TTOs	to take out (discharge medicines)
Tx	treatment
U&Es	urea and electrolytes
U/S	ultrasound
UC	ulcerative colitis
UTA	unable to attend
UTI	urinary tract infection

VD	venereal disease
VF	ventricular fibrillation
VQ scan	ventilation perfusion scan
VZIG	varicella zoster immune globulin
WBC	white blood cell/count
WD	withdrawn (or specially imported drugs)
XR	X-ray

Subject Index

Note: Page numbers followed by 'f' and 't' refer to figures and tables respectively